# BRAIN HEALTH FOR LIFE

*Beyond Pills, Politics, and Popular Diets*

# BRAIN HEALTH FOR LIFE

*Beyond Pills, Politics,*
*and Popular Diets*

## KAREN V. UNGER, M.S.W., Ed.D.
### WITH LuANNE H. CAVENDER, N.T.P.

PORTLAND • OREGON
INKWATERPRESS.COM

*Scan QR code for
more information
on this book.*

Cover and interior design by Masha Shubin
Edited by Holly Tri

Author Photographer: Diane Benjamin
Brain Aging © digitalista. BigStockPhoto.com
Brain Cloud © sellingpix. BigStockPhoto.com

Unger, Karen V.
   Brain health for life : beyond pills, politics, and
popular diets / by Karen V. Unger with LuAnne H.
Cavender.
   pages cm
   Includes bibliographical references.
   LCCN 2014912641
   ISBN 978-1-62901-154-7 (pbk.)
   ISBN 978-1-62901-131-8 (Kindle)
   ISBN 978-1-62901-156-1 (ePub)

   1. Brain--Aging--Prevention--Popular works. 2. Brain
--Care and hygiene--Popular works. 3. Nutrition--
Popular works.   I. Cavender, LuAnne H. II. Title.

QP376.U54 2014            612.8'2
                          QBI14-1866


Publisher: Inkwater Press | www.inkwaterpress.com

Paperback   ISBN-13 978-1-62901-154-7 | ISBN-10 1-62901-154-1
Kindle      ISBN-13 978-1-62901-155-4 | ISBN-10 1-62901-155-X
ePub        ISBN-13 978-1-62901-156-1 | ISBN-10 1-62901-156-8


Printed in the U.S.A.
All paper is acid free and meets all ANSI standards for archival quality paper.

3 5 7 9 10 8 6 4

The book will be of great value to those behavioral and physical health specialists who are working in the emerging area of integrated healthcare.

— Bob Nikkel, MSW, Board Member of the
Foundation for Excellence in Mental Health Care

… A great gift … straightforward, easy-to-read, and thoroughly comprehensive.

— Tanya J. Peterson, MS, NCC, author of
*Leave of Absence* and *My Life in a Nutshell*

Dr. Unger has written a straightforward book that covers all aspects of brain health including nutrition, supplementation and lifestyle choices. I will recommend *Brain Health for Life* to my clients as well as my friends and relatives.

— Joy Fitzpatrick Quinn, Master Trainer

… A concise resource for those looking to thwart cognitive decline and the numerous health challenges most Americans face today as a result of a nutritionally devoid diet.

— Dr. Kate Wiggin, N.D.

This is the first book to present exceedingly well-researched, clear and thorough information and recommendations to athletes for brain and body health. I expect it to be my essential desk reference for long-term physical and mental health.

— Robert A. Maestre, Master Swimmer

*To*
*Ian and Noah*

# Table of Contents

# Acknowledgements

I WOULD LIKE TO GRATEFULLY ACKNOWLEDGE THE CONTRIBUTION of LuAnne Cavender to the development of this book. As a certified Nutritional Therapy Practitioner with a background in biology and medical research, and two years of medical school, she has been an ever present and gracious consultant on nutrition and anatomy. LuAnne helped me define the parameters of the book's content and was always available to answer my questions and to point me to new resources. I could not have written this book without her.

I would like to also acknowledge the following people for their help and support in bringing this book to fruition. Each read a portion of the book and gave me helpful feedback that made me rethink and rewrite for greater clarity: Guin Hillman and Nancy Russell, members of my ever supportive book group, Barbara Summers for her continued encouragement, Ellen Houx for her attention to detail, Michael Moyhan for his interets and feedback, and Richard Minehard for being so scholarly and incisive in his comments. You have all been wonderful and I am so grateful to have you as friends.

I want to express my gratitude to my editor, Holly Tri, for her keen eye and helpful suggestions, to Masha Shubin for her stunning cover and interior design, and to Sean Jones and John Williams, the lead guys at Inkwater Press. You've all been extremely helpful and I appreciate your enthusiasm and expertise in bringing this book to publication.

# Introduction

TWO IMPORTANT DEVELOPMENTS ARE AFFECTING OUR BRAIN health. We are living longer and the incidences of dementia and Alzheimer's disease are increasing. Those of us who will be lucky enough to live into old age increasingly fear the onset of cognitive decline. We want our brains to last as long as our bodies, and although there are no cures for the diseases of the brain, we can live our lives now in a way that promotes brain health throughout our lifespans.

We assume a healthy body nourishes a healthy brain—and it's true. With advanced technology, like magnetic imaging (MRIs), cellular dye tagging, electron microscopy, and other technology, scientists can actually see what happens in individual brain cells. What makes a healthy body does make a healthy brain. Research is emerging that shows us how to have healthier bodies and healthier brains. This is what this book is about. Culling the numerous new books on diet and health, examining the scientific literature, and exploring the many sources of current information on the web, I have summarized the latest information on brain health in an understandable and concise way.

This book has been a journey that began when I read a 2009 report, "The State Of Health Of Clients Within The Extended Care Management Program," from the state agency Addictions and Mental Health in Oregon. The report indicated clients within the residential and hospital programs displayed the following conditions:

- One in eight had six different health related diagnoses other than mental health
- More than half had nervous system and sense organ related diseases
- More than a third had major cardiovascular diseases
- More than one in five had diabetes

Nationally, people with a severe mental illness die 25 years earlier than the general population. These statistics reflect the health conditions of adults within the mental health system. Their poor health creates an enormous burden on the physical healthcare system, and the reduction in quality of life for the patients is tragic. An intervention that promotes healthier clients and reduces healthcare costs is critical.

There is a growing body of evidence that links mental health and brain function to proper nutrition. As the American diet has deteriorated, due to the prevalence of fast food, processed food, and genetically modified food, nutritional deficiencies that correlate with mental disorders such as depression, schizophrenia, and bipolar disorder have become more common. Appropriate and adequate nutrients are essential to the physical structure of the brain and greatly influence its normal functioning.

Many studies link an individual's psychiatric diagnosis to a lack of specific nutrients. Physicians can combat particular symptoms of the mental illness with dietary supplements. However, this level of specificity requires extensive assessment and monitoring by professionals. A more generalized and feasible approach would be to promote an individual's food intake to provide the nutrients commonly needed by all brains for normal development and functioning.

When I read "The State Of Health Of Clients Within The Extended Care Management Program," I had been working for the State of Oregon to develop programs to improve the educational opportunities for clients within the system. After I read the report I contacted several mental health agencies with residential facilities to set up programs to promote clients' physical health and, at the same time, improve their brain health. Although there was great interest, the programs did not receive funding. However, I was very intrigued and continued my exploration of the correlation between physical health and brain health. As I broadened my knowledge, I decided to broaden my focus to the general population.

About the same time, I met LuAnne Cavender, a Nutritional Therapy Practitioner with an extensive background in the health sciences and functional medicine. We worked together to develop the residential programs and she has been an invaluable consultant to me as I have written this book. LuAnne is a virtual fountain of knowledge about health and nutrition. She keeps current in her field and has been instrumental in shaping the content of this book and guiding my research.

As a social worker and educator, I have developed programs, completed research projects, and written extensivley on issues related to mental health at Sargent College of Allied Health Professions, Boston University in Boston; the Research & Training Center for Children's Mental Health at the Louis de la Parte Florida Mental Health Institute, University of South Florida in Tampa; and the Program for Community Development and Integration at the University of Arizona in Tucson. I am currently a research associate professor at the Graduate School of Eduction, Portland State University in Portland, Oregon.

As I continued my research, I realized there were numerous books on diet advocating many different approaches. But the questions that motivated me were, how did food affect the brain? How could we keep our brains healthy and functioning into old age? This book has evolved to answer those questions. Armed with this information, we can make informed choices and do our best to live out our lives with all of our faculties intact.

# Down the Primrose Path

# CHAPTER I

# Politics and Your Pantry

My grandparents emigrated from Sweden in the early 1900s and homesteaded on the North Dakota prairie, where they raised five children on a small farm. Conditions were harsh and the labor never let up, but the lifestyle and food made for strong, healthy bodies. There was fresh, whole milk from the cows and meat from the steers and hogs. The chickens provided both meat and eggs. A large garden and a small orchard supplied fresh vegetables and fruit. Picking berries, chokecherries, and wild plums added variety to their diet and their routine. The cattle grazed on the prairie grass in the summer and fed on hay and silage during the winter. The chickens scratched in the barnyard for seeds and bugs, and their diet was supplemented with grain. The hogs were fed kitchen leftovers and grain. Butter was churned from the rich cream given by the milking cows, and cooking fat came from rendering the hog fat into lard.

My grandparents fed no antibiotics or growth hormones to their livestock. The fertilizer for the garden and crops came from the barnyard. Food for the winter, including fruits and vegetables canned by my grandmother, was stored in the root cellar. Cash came from selling grain, eggs, and sour cream that fermented in milk cans, and from bringing the hogs and cattle to market. The water came from the family well. The farm diet included very little sugar, no diet sodas, no trans fats, and no processed food. Lights went out early in the evening because work started early in the morning. My aunts and uncles thrived and all lived into their late 80s and 90s. My uncle John set the record by living to age 104. My own father lived to age 99. There was little evidence of heart disease, diabetes, cognitive decline, or Alzheimer's in any of them. One aunt died of bowel cancer at 89.

My grandparents' small farm, like most of the others throughout that rural county, was sold in the sixties. The land went to another farmer who uses the land for grazing. The farmhouse was moved to town and the barn and outbuildings fell into ruin. Commercial farming by corporations is not feasible on this land; it is not productive enough and the weather is harsh and unpredictable. It has been saved from the fate of industrialized farming and the overuse of commercial fertilizers for growing crops that strip the land of its natural fecundity. There are no huge chicken pens or feed lots that deprive the birds and animals of a decent life. It's just open land for grazing, preserving many of native prairie grasses and the natural wildlife.

But life has changed greatly since my grandparents' time. Our current diet and lifestyle spawns preventable diseases such as cardiovascular disease, strokes, autoimmune disorders, obesity and diabetes, Alzheimer's and other brain disorders.

Consider this:

- Sixty-nine percent of adults in the US are overweight or obese.
- Rates of "extreme" obesity have risen from 1.4% thirty years ago to 6.3% today, an increase of 350%.
- Over 8% of the entire country has diabetes. Eighty percent of those are overweight.
- One in four deaths is caused by heart disease, the number one cause of death in the US.
- Although cancer rates are declining, it is still the second leading cause of death.
- Stroke is the third leading cause of death.
- The sixth leading cause of death is Alzheimer's disease.

- Obesity-related medical costs total 147 billion dollars a year, 10 percent of all annual medical spending.

In September 2010 the United Nations declared that, for the first time in human history, chronic, non-communicable diseases, such as heart disease, cancer, and diabetes, pose a greater health burden worldwide than infectious diseases, contributing to 35 million deaths annually. A report from the National Cancer Institute states, "For more than 30 years, excess weight, insufficient physical activity, and an unhealthy diet have been second only to tobacco as preventable causes of death and diseases in the United States." How did we get here?

## Food Politics

We want to believe our federal government, the agencies of the federal government, professional organizations, and food producers have bringing the best possible food products to us, the consumers, as their highest priority. Although their mandates and mission statements may reflect this priority, there are many variables, such as profits and politics, that muddy the waters. Professional organizations for the meat, chicken, dairy, soy, and sugar industries, as well as organizations representing the nutrition, health, and pharmaceutical industries, have often put their financial and political goals ahead of our health. The United States Department of Agriculture (USDA), specifically, and the agencies under their administration, such as the Department of Health and Human Services (DHHS), the National Institute of Health (NIH), the Food and Drug Administration (FDA), among others, have competing interests, cherished beliefs, and many constituents to mollify.

In the introduction to *Food, Inc.*, the editor, Karl Weber, notes, "Our nation's food supply is now controlled by a handful of corporations that often put profit ahead of consumer health, the livelihood of the American farmer, the safety of workers, and our natural environment. Furthermore, it is done with the "consent of our government's regulatory agencies, the US Department of Agriculture (USDA) and the Food and Drug Administration (FDA)." (p. vii)

Marion Nestle is a respected nutritionist and author of several books on nutrition. She was a committee chair on the first *Dietary Guidelines for Americans* working for the Public Health Service. She writes in her book *Food Politics: How the Food Industry Influences Nutrition and Health*:

> Food companies will make and market any product that sells, regardless of its nutritional value or effects on health. ... The ways in which the food industry practices distort what Americans are told about nutrition—and compromise food choices—raises serious issues that are worth consideration by anyone concerned about nutrition and health. (p. vii)

Eric Schlosser, in his meticulously researched 2001 book, *Fast Food Nation: The Dark Side of the All-American Meal*, describes how the food industry-friendly policies of the federal government have affected our food supply, creating low-wage jobs, unsafe working conditions, and lack of oversight for food and worker safety. Although more than a decade has passed since its publication, Schlosser notes in the Afterword of the 2012 edition that the founding fathers:

> ... If they were alive today, like Upton Sinclair they would be amazed by the monopolies and monopsonies that now dominate the American economy, by the corruption of government officials and the wide disparities of wealth. The food industry needs to become part of a larger movement ... that demands not only healthy food but also a living wage and a safe workplace for every single American. (p. 275)

When the USDA was established in 1900, its mission was to (1) "insure a sufficient and reliable food supply" and (2) "provide general and comprehensive information to citizens." That mandate continues today but has had an ambiguous effect. Promoting agriculture and agricultural products and providing information about food and food products are often at cross-purposes with each other. The kind of information disseminated to consumers by the USDA often affects the sale of agriculture products. What might be good for the consumer may not be good for agriculture and what might be good for the consumer may not necessarily promote the products.

The development of soy protein is an example of these competing priorities. Hailed as a revolutionary healthful alternative food source, it is in reality a highly processed product that has questionable value for consumers. Although it is an extremely profitable product for the soy industry, as a byproduct of the extraction of soy oil, soy protein is basically a waste product dressed up as "health food." Soy protein now appears in many foods, from protein bars and hamburger to ice cream.

To promote soy products, soybean producers pay a mandatory assessment of one-half to one percent of the net market price of soybeans to develop and strengthen domestic and foreign markets for its products. Like many other agricultural products, soy has a strong lobby behind it. The lobbyists are former legislators, agricultural committee members, marketing experts, and nutritionists.

This lobby has been very effective. In late 1999 the Food and Drug Administration approved a health claim that permits soy processors to label many soy products with the phrase, "Diets low in saturated fat and cholesterol that include 25 grams of soy protein a day may reduce the risk of heart disease." The FDA, in approving this claim, ignored contrary evidence, including recommendations by their own scientists at the National Center for Toxicology.

Many of the lobbyists for the beef and soy industries, as well as others, have held previous positions in agriculture or related industries that directly affect the formation of policies and recommendations for food and nutrition guidelines. According to Mark Bittman, a *New York Times* columnist, half the people who developed the food pyramid were or had been linked to agribusiness. An example of the close relationship between agriculture production and federal regulators is a recent appointee to the Food and Drug Administration. As an attorney, this government official has held high positions with the USDA and was an assistant to the FDA commissioner before he was employed by the Monsanto law offices. As one of Monsanto's attorneys, he led the firm's food and drug law practice and worked to gain FDA approval of Monsanto's recombinant bovine somatotropin (rBST). rBST has been banned in Canada, Australia, New Zealand, Japan, Israel, and the European Union since 2000, because it causes "severe and unnecessary pain, suffering and distress" for cows. He is now the FDA's Deputy Commissioner for Foods and Veterinary Medicine.

Other means of influence are less visible. Food companies provide information and funds for professional societies, conferences, and meetings. Corporate donors provide funding for academic departments at colleges and universities through research grants, scholarships, equipment, facilities, and buildings. Corporations also sponsor professional journals, including nutritional journals and medical journals. Recipients of this financial support benefit financially and professionally, and although it does not necessarily mean they will support or endorse the corporation's products, it makes one wonder how free they are to put forth ideas that run counter to their sponsors' interests. To counter this impression at the academic level, many colleges and universities now have disclosure policies.

Organizations that appear to promote healthy food and healthy living also have practices that call into question their values. The American Heart Association (AHA) proposed a program in 1994 that would, for a fee, endorse products as "heart healthy." The initial cost for this seal of approval to the product company was $2,500, with an annual renewal fee of $650, and more for exclusive rights. The practice continues today. The AHA defends the program, although the "heart healthy" foods would raise most educated consumer's eyebrows. Campbell's V8 Splash, for example, endorsed by the AHA for its low level of saturated fat and cholesterol, contains high fructose corn syrup, 10 percent fruit and vegetable concentrates, artificial coloring, and the artificial sweetener sucralose.

Members of the American Dietetic Association (ADA) are important contributors to the Dietary Guideline Alliance that developed the *Food Pyramid* and *Food Plate*. It's a professional association made up of nutritionists who are credentialed as registered dietitians. The ADA has partnerships with food companies or trade organizations that fund their programs and contribute to their research efforts. Corporate sponsors/partners include PepsiCo, Coca-Cola, Mars, Hershey's, General Mills, and others. Again, the influence of the corporate sponsors is pervasive and sometimes subtle. For example, the credentialing arm of the ADA has approved a program created by the Coca-Cola Company Beverage Institute for Health & Wellness. This program will review the "urban myths" about the safety of fluoride, sugar, artificial colors, and artificial sweeteners. Registered dietitians who participate in the program will earn registered continuing professional education credits.

The ADA is currently promoting legislation, with the support of their sponsors, Coca-Cola and Hershey's, to prohibit Naturalpaths, Nutritional Counselors, Liscensed Nutritionists, and other nutritional professionals from giving advice on nutrition and food. It would effectivley promote a monoploy for the registered dietitians and, essentially, limit consumer access to alternative philosophies, assessments, and treatment. The standards and requirements for the practice of nutritionists are most often broader than the standards for dietitians, but this type of legislation would allow only licensed dietitians to legally offer nutritional services, including performing nutritional assessments and nutrition monitoring, counseling, and evaluation—skills that currently fall under the purview and practice of a nutritionist.

# The Food Pyramid

Since 1980, by law, the federal government must publish the *Dietary Guidelines for Americans* every five years. The National

Nutrition Monitoring and Related Research Act of 1990 requires the secretaries of the United States Department of Agriculture and the Department of Health and Human Services to publish a joint report that contains nutritional and dietary guidelines for the general public. It must be based on "the preponderance of scientific and medical knowledge current at the time of publication." The USDA and DHHS appoint a Dietary Guidelines Advisory Committee of prominent experts in nutrition and health to review the scientific and medical knowledge current at the time and recommend to the secretaries of USDA and DHHS any revisions to the previous guidelines they feel are warranted.

The USDA, in fulfilling its mandate "to provide general and comprehensive information to citizens" has been issuing guides or dietary guidelines throughout its history. The first USDA food guide, *How to Select Foods*, appeared in 1917, followed by various revisions. In the early 1940s, with the discovery of vitamins and minerals, the food guides took a sharper focus to emphasize the nutritional content of food choices.

*The Basic Four* was introduced in 1958, responding to new demographic information from reports of malnutrition throughout the country. It included four food groups: milk, meat, vegetables and fruit, and bread and cereal. *The Basic Four* established minimum levels of daily servings to ensure a healthy intake of necessary nutrients.

*Dietary Goals*, the next revision, occurred in 1977 and responded to reports that linked diet and chronic diseases. The new goals recommended that carbohydrate consumption be increased and fat, saturated fat, cholesterol, sugar, and salt consumption be decreased. By recommending eating less fat, saturated fat, cholesterol, sugar, and salt, the latter five were implicated in the increase of the chronic diseases. After *Dietary Goals* was issued, the meat, dairy, egg, and other mentioned food producers were outraged and lobbied to have the language of the guidelines revised to be more favorable to their industries. The changes were made.

*Healthy People*, issued by the Department of Health, Education, and Welfare (HEW), the precursor to DHHS, followed two years later. The emphasis again was on preventing disease. Consumers were urged to eat more complex carbohydrates, more fish, and more poultry, but to eat less red meat, fat, salt, and sugar. *Healthy People* also recommended consumers pay attention to the quality of the processed foods they were eating.

*Dietary Guidelines for Americans* was issued one year later as a response to the passage of the 1980 law mandating a review of the *Guidelines*. This document was an effort to placate the industries that felt they had been slighted in the previous 1977 document. The wording was changed from "eat less" red meat, fat, salt, and sugar to the more innocuous language "avoid too much."

The *Dietary Guidelines for Americans* was revised in 1985, 1988, and 1990 to again address the concern of various food industries. The *Food Guide Pyramid* finally replaced the *Guidelines* in 1992. However, an earlier version (1991), The *Eating Right Pyramid,* was not distributed because the meat and dairy industries objected to the placement of their products towards the top, where the proportions were smaller. The *Food Guide Pyramid* addressed their concerns by changing the number of recommended servings.

The *Food Guide Pyramid* remained the nutritional guide for the next two decades, continuing to emphasize a high carbohydrate, low-fat diet. The Pyramid recommended 6 to 11 daily servings of potatoes, pasta, bread, rice, or corn, foods that lead directly to high blood pressure, type 2 diabetes, and obesity. Limiting fatty food and oils, along with meat, butter, and cheese, which we now know are healthy choices, was also recommended. Most recently, a new approach has been taken to make the dietary recommendations more understandable. Enter *MyPlate*. *MyPlate* shows a plate with the food divided into four quadrants: grains 30%, vegetables 30%, fruit 20%, and protein 20%. No fat is pictured.

What the food pyramid and the food plate fail to take into consideration, however, is the latest research on the importance of good fat in our diets, particularly from naturally raised red meat, fish, poultry, eggs, and whole fat dairy products, including butter. The primary emphasis continues to be on grain and cereal products, which research shows contribute to the obesity epidemic.

Our eating habits and our weight have changed over the years. Whether the changes are caused by the continued revisions of dietary choices by the USDA, our changing lifestyles, or the emphasis on certain products by food producers and their advertisers is anybody's guess. What we do know is that today two-thirds of the United States population is overweight or obese.

Our increased consumption of certain food products may help explain this weight gain. Based on the *Per Capita Consumption of Major Food Commodities: 1980–2010*, our consumption of flour and cereal products has increased 52 pounds per person in the last ten years. We consume 16 more pounds of caloric sweeteners per person each year than we did ten years ago. Although the federal government acknowledges the explosion of the number of overweight and obese citizens and the incidences of both type 1 and type 2 diabetes, it continues to ignore the role that carbohydrates and sugar play in this trend and the benefits of good fat.

The *2005 Report of the Dietary Guidelines Advisory Committee* states:

> The major way to keep saturated fat low is to limit one's intake of animal fats (such as those in cheese, milk, butter, ice cream, and other full-fat dairy products; fatty meat; bacon and sausage; and poultry skin and fat). ... To limit dietary intake of cholesterol, one needs to limit the intake of eggs and organ meats especially, as well as limit the intake of meat, shellfish, and poultry and dairy products that contain fat. (p. 5)

The report also concludes that there is no relationship between total carbohydrate intake (minus fiber) and the incidence of either type 1 or type 2 diabetes. Regarding sugar, they say the evidence suggests a positive association between the consumption of sugar-sweetened beverages and weight gain.

# Food and Your Brain

We need to consider the latest research when choosing what to eat. *MyPlate* and the accompanying information on the website have updated the *Food Guide Pyramid* to help us choose healthy, nutritious food, but the emphasis continues to be on grains and carbohydrates, which we know contribute to chronic, preventable diseases. Consumption of healthy fat as an important component of a complete diet, particularly for the brain, is discouraged.

The popularity of and addiction to fast foods and processed foods containing excess amounts of fat, sugar, and salt also contribute to the national crisis of rising obesity and disease. As our nation ages and we continue with our current diet and lifestyle, preventable diseases, including Alzheimer's and dementia, are going to become a national crisis.

Considerable evidence points to food choices and lifestyle as key to defending our brains from dementia and Alzheimer's. Diet, mental and physical exercise, stress reduction, and social engagement may all delay the onset of dementia for many people. A recent National Institute of Health consensus panel reported, "Many studies of healthy lifestyle habits—including diet, physical activity and cognitive engagement—are providing insights into the prevention of cognitive decline and Alzheimer's disease." (p. 7) Evidence from the *MacArthur Study of Successful Aging* explained that to prevent Alzheimer's disease, lifestyle and diet were two major predictors of physical and mental health. Our genes, the third factor, account for only a third of the equation. A lifestyle and diet that promotes brain health not only strengthens neurons and postpones mental decline, it also improves memory and brain efficiency almost immediately.

# Back to the Farm?

Wouldn't it be wonderful if we could return to the small farms like my grandparents' farm? Naturally raised food and livestock, homegrown vegetables and wild fruit, and plenty of exercise and fresh air would promote health for both our bodies and our minds. Although small farm life has some appeal, few of us would choose to go back, and we are left to make difficult choices in our modern world. To maintain good brain health, we do need to make changes from eating highly processed foods, too many carbohydrates, too much sugar, and too few good fats, to the diet of our grandparents'. We need to be cautious about the advice of the federal government and affiliated agencies and make our own informed choices. We need to resist the appeal of super palatable foods and supersized portions. We can choose to eat healthier food. In doing so, we can decrease our chances of getting dementia, Alzheimer's, diabetes, heart disease, cancer, and other debilitating diseases. We cannot go back to the farm, and we may not live to be 104 as my uncle did, but we can take responsibility for our health.

# CHAPTER 2

# Fast Food, Processed Food, and GMOs

## Fast Food

Foods containing high amounts of fat, sugar, and salt sell like hotcakes. Potato chips, cookies, cheese fries, and Buffalo wings, and main meals slathered and marinated with sauces stimulate the pleasure centers of our brain and function like opiates. Opiates are chemicals produced by the brain and create effects similar to those created by morphine and heroin. "Stimulating the opioid circuitry with food drives us to eat," says Dr. David Kessler in his book *The End of Overeating: Taking Control of the Insatiable American Appetite.* (p. 37) He calls these foods "super palatable." Like the cravings for street drugs, the more fat, sugar, and salt we eat, the more fat, sugar, and salt we crave. Our brains are being rewired to anticipate and seek out the pleasure that comes from eating super palatable foods.

Oreos, America's favorite cookies, are an example. A new study by Dr. Joseph Schroeder from Connecticut College found Oreos to be as addictive as cocaine or morphine. When the cookies were eaten by laboratory rats, whose brains function similar to ours, they triggered the production of the brains' natural opiates. The cookies activated more neurons in the rats' pleasure centers than cocaine or morphine. Oreos are not alone in their appeal to our brains. Whole industries have sprung up to design food that is super palatable and highly appealing. Nowhere is this more prevalent than in the fast food industry.

Fast foods have become a diet staple for many people. Although nutritionists recommend eating at fast food restaurants no more than once a month, one in four Americans eats out every day. Morgan Spurlock, director of the documentary *Supersize Me*, notes that 43% of those eat at McDonalds, home of the supersized almost everything. Although McDonalds has discontinued their supersized drink, at 42 ounces (6 ounces short of three quarts), with 48 teaspoons of sugar, most of their food items contain huge amounts of sugar, fat, and salt.

## Fast Food and the National Health Crisis

According to government statistics, Americans over-consume added sugars and discretionary/added fats and oils and under-consume fruit, vegetables, whole grains, and dairy. Tomatoes and potatoes account for almost half of the total vegetable consumption. Few dark green or orange-colored vegetables are eaten. If we were aware of what was in our food, we might make better choices. Fortunately, the regulations on food labeling give us some clues. Here is the calorie content in some favorite fast foods:

- McDonald's Big Mac: 540 calories
- Burger King Whopper: 670 calories
- Taco Bell Nachos Bell Grande: 770 calories
- Dairy Queen Onion Rings: 360 calories
- Popeye's Regular Cole Slaw: 260 calories
- Wendy's Large Frosty: 540 calories
- Dunkin Donut's Iced Carmel Latte: 450 calories

Not only do fast foods contain large amount of calories, they also contain some unexpected ingredients. Here is a sample of some additives:

- Eggs and premium egg blend in egg sandwiches: glycerin, dimethylpolysiloxane, and calcium silicate
- McNuggets: bones, carcasses, and leftover chicken parts—pink sludge (McDonalds disputes this report and says nuggets "are made from USDA inspected boneless white meat chicken")
- Tacos from Taco Bell: formerly accused of serving only 36% beef in its beef dishes, the meat comes preprocessed in sheets
- McRib: 70 ingredients made by restructured meat technology, including tripe, heart, scalded stomach, pork trimmings, azodicarbonamide, and more

Eight different brands of fast food hamburgers were analyzed, and investigators found the meat content ranged from 2.1% to 14.8% (median 12.1%). Electron microscopy showed skeletal muscle, connective tissue, blood vessels, peripheral nerve, adipose tissue, plant material, and cartilage and bone in the meat. Two also contained intracellular parasites (Sarcocystis). Approximately half the weight of the hamburgers was water.

Many products have sauces to dip meat into, and according to the USDA, it is acceptable for the sauces to contain "30 or more fly eggs per 100 grams" and "1 or more maggots per 100 grams." Although salad seems like a good alternative, it is often coated with propylene glycol, a product used in antifreeze and sexual lubricants, to keep the leaves crisp. Chemicals to improve the taste and appearance of food, including methyl 2-pyridyl ketone or ethyl 3-hydroxybutanoate, can be listed as "natural flavors" on the product labels, including those products identified as organic.

The deli case is not the best alternative to preparing meals at home either. A recent trip to a national grocery chain to purchase two side dishes, broccoli raisin salad and Northwest potato salad, was instructive. Between the two salads, they contained 55 ingredients. In addition to recognizable food items and flavorings, there were three forms of sugar, three different food colorings, (FD&C Blue #1, FD&C Red #4 and FD&C yellow #5), sodium phosphate, sodium erythorbate, sodium nitrate, sodium benzoate, potassium sorbate, and xanthan gum. Most of these ingredients are harmless in the amounts used in foods, but may cause reactions in people who are sensitive to dyes and additives.

With our addiction to fast foods containing unhealthy amounts of sugar, fat, and salt, obesity is a nationwide health problem. Obesity increases the chances of developing clogged arteries, high blood pressure, type 2 diabetes, and some forms of cancer. How much fast food is too much? The USDA reports that one or more fast food meal per week is associated with obesity.

Normal BMI (body mass index), a measure to determine one's body fat percentage, is between 18.5 and 24.99. The rate of "extreme" obesity (BMI over 40, or 100 pounds over the ideal weight) has grown by 350% in the last 30 years, from 1.4 to 6.0%. Among children and teens (2- to 19-year-olds), more than 5.1% of males and 4.7% of females are now morbidly or extremely obese.

Obesity rates between men and women are similar. Rates for Baby Boomers (45- to 64-year-olds) are higher than both seniors and young adults. More adults without a high school education are obese than those with high school graduation or college. Income is also a discriminating factor. People who earn less than $25,000 per year are more likely to be obese.

According to "F as in Fat: How Obesity Threatens America's Future," published in 2012 by the Robert Wood Johnson Foundation and the Trust for America's Health, half the adults in America will be obese by 2030 if present trends continue. Fortunately, the 2013 "F as in Fat" report finds adult obesity rates remained level in every state except one, Arkansas. However, obesity is a national problem. Thirteen states now have obesity rates above 30%. Forty-one states have rates of at least 25%. In 1980 no state was above 15%. Child obesity rates, as of 2011–2012, have not changed significantly since 2003–2004 and remain at approximately 17%.

# Food Labels

According to US labeling laws, food producers must list the nutrients in the food and their "Percent Daily Value" (%DV). Percent Daily Value tells the percent of the recommended daily intake in a serving of that product. The rule of thumb is 20%DV or more is high and 5% or less is low. Read the labels for calorie and nutrient content in processed, packaged, and canned foods. Whole foods and animal products have a different kind of label that tells where and how they were grown or raised.

**Organic foods.** The federal government sets standards for labeling fresh food. Foods labeled organic must be free of potentially harmful pesticides, herbicides, chemical fertilizers, sewage sludge, artificial hormones, antibiotics, and genetically modified organisms (GMOs). The food must not have been processed using irradiation, chemical food additives, or industrial solvents. Products made with 95 to 100% certified organic foods may display the USDA Organic seal on their packages.

**Made with organic.** If a product is "made with" organic products, at least 70% of the product is certified organic. The remaining 30% may not be.

**Natural.** The term "natural" applies to foods that are minimally processed and free of synthetic preservatives: artificial sweeteners, colors, flavors, and other artificial additives; hydrogenated oils; stabilizers; and emulsifiers. Most foods labeled natural are not subject to government controls beyond the regulations and health codes that apply to all foods. The term "natural" is not regulated except for meat and poultry.

Natural meat and poultry must be free of artificial colors, flavors, sweeteners, preservatives, and ingredients. These products must be minimally processed in a method that does not fundamentally change them. The label must also explain the use of the term natural, such as "no artificial ingredients." A "natural" label on meat and poultry does not refer to how the animals were raised.

**Healthy.** Healthy, defined by regulation, means the product must meet certain criteria that limit the amounts of fat, saturated fat, cholesterol, and sodium, and contain specific amounts of vitamins, minerals, or other beneficial nutrients.

## Effects of Fast Food on Health

The effects of fast food on health are sobering. The International Study of Asthma and Allergies in Childhood (ISAAC) involved more than 100 countries and nearly 2 million children. A link was found between three or more servings of fast food a week and the severity of allergic asthma, eczema, and rhinitis among children in the developed world. On the other hand, fruit seemed to be protective for all three conditions.

"Every day in the United States," according to Eric Schlosser, author of *Fast Food Nation*, "roughly 200,000 people are sickened by a food borne disease, 900 are hospitalized and 14 die." He also explains that many foodborne pathogens can cause long-term ailments, such as heart disease, inflammatory bowel disease, neurological problems, autoimmune disorders, and kidney damage. Other writers make the point that the animals people eat may actually be sick from malnutrition and diseases. The Center for Disease Control (CDC) reports that more than a quarter of the American population suffers a bout of food poisoning each year. Most cases are never reported to authorities or properly diagnosed.

Eating commercial baked goods (cakes, doughnuts, croissants, etc.) and fast food (hamburgers, hot dogs, pizza, etc.) is linked not only to physical ailments, but to depression as well. People who eat fast food are 51% more likely to develop depression, according to a study of 8,964 participants from the University of Las Palmas de Gran Canaria and the University of Granada. The more fast food eaten, the greater the risk of depression.

# Processed Foods

## Food Processing Gone Awry

Any food that is not in its natural form is processed in some way. Our grocery stores are stacked to the ceilings with processed food labeled "heart healthy," "natural," "low-fat," "cholesterol free," or "high in vitamins and minerals." Don't be fooled. In many cases, the natural ingredients have been taken out and replaced with "enriched" or "fortified" food product, and numerous unnatural ingredients have been added, some the body may not recognize as food.

Food processing has been with us for millenniums. Dried, canned, pickled, or fermented foods have been prepared by our forbearers, indigenous people, and early civilizations to aid in digestion or for preservation for later use. Using fresh, whole ingredients, millers, bakers, cheese makers, distillers, and homemakers processed grains and animal products into nutritious food that was delicious and digestible and freshly made or that would keep for weeks or months. Preservation or processing allowed them to have a varied diet throughout the year. Somewhere along the line, however, things went a little off. Soybeans are a good example.

**Soy products: natural processing vs. industrial processing.** Soy and soy products have been sold to the American people as a health-promoting food that prevents diseases. One of the advertised claims is that the Chinese have consumed soy for millenniums and therefore soy must be healthy. However, the consumption of soybeans by Asian countries has been largely exaggerated. In their raw form, soybeans contain large quantities of antinutrients. Antinutrients include enzyme inhibitors that block the action of enzymes needed for protein digestion and the uptake of amino acids. Soybeans also contain high concentrations of phytates, which prevent the absorption of calcium, magnesium, iron, and zinc. To make the soybean more palatable, the Chinese processed it by naturally fermenting it, making miso (fermented soy paste), shoyu (soy sauce), tofu (soy curd), nattō (fermented soy cheese), and tempeh made by a natural culturing and controlled fermentation.

In the United States we seldom consume soybeans in their traditionally processed form. Instead, we process soybeans by using hexane or other solvents to remove the oil (which can be sold as cooking oil or oil to be added to other processed foods) and then take what's leftover (defatted soy flour) and either combine it with other proteins to make animal feed or wash it with water to create soy protein concentrate. Soy protein concentrate becomes the source for two forms of soy that are even more processed: TVP, or textured soy protein is produced through a process called extrusion (more about this process later). The other product, soy protein isolate (SPI), is produced by making the soy protein concentrate more solubilized and is an ingredient in low-fat soy milk.

SPI is produced through a high temperature process that forms nitrates and a toxin called lysinoalanine. Flavorings are added, including MSG, to improve the taste. The end products are used widely in school lunch programs, in commercial baked goods, in soy milk and diet beverages, and in fast food products. These foods create unintended consequences. In the article "Newest Research On Why You Should Avoid Soy," authors Fallon and Enig state:

> In feeding experiments, the use of SPI increased requirement for vitamins E, K, D and B12 and created deficiency symptoms of calcium, magnesium, manganese, molybdenum, copper, iron and zinc. Phytic acid remaining in these soy products greatly inhibits zinc and iron absorption; test animals fed SPI develop enlarged organs, particularly the pancreas and thyroid gland, and increased fatty acids in the liver. (p. 2)

When producers of SPI sought FDA approval, there was strong opposition by scientists, including a report by the British government that warned against potential adverse effects. Soy products have been granted GRAS (generally recognized as safe) status only as a cardboard binder. Today the sale of all soy products as food or a food additive is subject to premarket approval procedures by the FDA.

On the other hand, proponents of soy have gained considerable attention, claiming soy improves the risk factors for cardiovascular disease and has many other health benefits. Contrary to these beliefs, scientists Sacks, Lichtenstein, Van Horn, and others found soy protein isolate had:

> No significant effects on HDL cholesterol, triglycerides, lipoprotein (a), or blood pressure were evident. Among 19 studies of soy isoflavones, the average effect on LDL cholesterol and other lipid risk factors was nil. Soy protein and isoflavones have not been shown to lessen vasomotor symptoms of menopause, and results are mixed with regard to soy's ability to slow postmenopausal bone loss. The efficacy and safety of soy isoflavones for preventing or treating cancer of the breast, endometrium, and prostate are not established; evidence from clinical trials is meager and cautionary with regard to a possible adverse effect. For this reason, use of isoflavone supplements in food or pills is not recommended.

**Cold breakfast cereals.** Cold breakfast cereals, another example of processed food, start out well enough with whole grains, but then things take a turn. Grains are mixed with water, processed into slurry, and placed into a machine called an extruder where they are heated to a high temperature. The slurry is subjected to high pressure, which shapes it into o's or stars or whatever shape is required as they are extruded. In the case of corn flakes, frosted flakes, etc., the corn is broken down into small grits and steam cooked under 20 pounds per square inch of pressure. The nutritious germ with its essential fats is removed so the product will not go rancid and the shelf life will not be shortened. After shaping, the cereal may be coated with vitamins, minerals, sweeteners, flavors, fruit juices, food colors, or preservatives. Sugar and oil is sprayed on the finished product to make it crisp and to prevent it from becoming soggy in milk.

The extrusion process damages much of the grain's nutrients and alters the proteins. Many of the health benefits claimed for breakfast cereals rely on the fortification of nutrients rather than the nutrients from the natural ingredients. The high heat may alter the molecular structure of the proteins and turn them into toxins. An unpublished study from the University of Michigan in Ann Arbor found that rats fed water and the cardboard box the cereal came in lived longer than rats fed water and cornflakes. Before they died, the cornflakes-fed rats had fits, bit each other, and went into convulsions. Autopsies revealed dysfunction of the pancreas, liver, and kidneys, and degeneration of the nerves of the spine, all signs of insulin shock. There are no published studies about the effects of manufactured cereals on humans. However, because they are fortified with synthetic nutrients, the USDA claims they are as healthy as the grains they are made from.

**Nature's perfect food: milk.** Raw, organic milk contains vital nutrients and fats that make it one of nature's most perfect foods. It contains casein proteins, whey proteins, milk sugar, 12 minerals, 5 acids, and vitamins and enzymes. It has the ideal ratio of omega-6 to omega-3 fatty acids: two to three.

Processed milk loses much of its vital nutrients. Pasteurization, the heating of milk to a certain temperature for a period of time to kill harmful bacteria, also alters the amino acids of lysine and tyrosine, reducing the impact of the complex proteins available in raw milk. Vitamin C loss may exceed 50%, and the loss of other water-soluble vitamins may be as high as 80%. Vitamin B12 is destroyed and the availability of the minerals calcium, chloride, magnesium, and others are reduced. Pasteurization also destroys the enzymes in milk. To restore the healthful benefits of milk, Vitamin D is added. Pasteurization also alters the molecular structure of the proteins of the milk, enabling them to pass through the walls of the intestines, creating leaky gut syndrome. Most milk products are made from pasteurized milk.

Pasteurization began in the 1920s in response to tuberculosis, infant diarrhea, and other diseases caused by poor animal nutrition and dirty production methods. Today, with milking machines, refrigeration, and sterile storage and transportation methods, there is little chance for the milk to become contaminated. However, the USDA warns that unpasteurized milk can pose a serious health problem and has limited its distribution across state lines.

Most milk found in traditional supermarkets is also homogenized. Homogenization is done to prevent the milk fat (cream) from rising to the top of the milk. Instead, the milk is forced under extreme pressure through tiny holes, altering the fat globules and distributing them more evenly throughout the milk. The reshaped fat molecules more readily pass through the gut wall, possibly accounting for the increased allergies to dairy products that are prevalent today. In the case of low-fat or reduced-fat milk, the fat is removed and used to make other commercial products, such as cheese and yogurt.

There are other issues with the commercial milk supply. Genetically engineered cow hormones are injected into dairy cows to increase their milk production. Recombinant bovine growth hormone (rBGH), recombinant bovine somatotropin (rBST), and insulin growth factor-1 (IGF-1) increase milk production by about 10%, but they are also absorbed from the milk into our digestive systems and have been linked to breast, colon, and prostate cancers.

But there is more. Recently, 2013, the International Dairy Food Association and the National Milk Producers Federation have petitioned the FDA to permit the alteration of the definition of milk to include chemical sweeteners such as aspartame and sucralose without including them on the ingredient label. The organizations are concerned that the sweeteners listed on the label would sidetrack consumers and cause them to overlook the nutritional value of the milk.

## Chemicals in Processed Foods

In addition to altering whole food, food processors also add ingredients. Many ingredients, such as food dyes that are linked to serious illnesses, from gastrointestinal disorders to cancer, have been banned in other countries. For example, Citrus Red #2, Yellow #5, and Yellow #6 have been banned in Norway and Finland. Blue #1 and Blue #2 have been banned in Norway, Finland, and France. Red #3 and Red #4 have been banned in the US for topical use, but can be added to our food and beverages. Carmel colorings in colas and chocolate flavored products are linked to various cancers.

Brominated vegetable oil, used as an emulsifier, affects the thyroid and is banned in over 100 countries. Potassium Bromate is used in baking pastries and breads and is banned in many European countries, Canada, China, and other countries. Butylated hydroxyanisole and butylated hydroxytoluene, used to prevent cereals and meats from becoming rancid, is banned in the United Kingdom, many other European countries, and Japan. Azodicarbonamide, used to bleach flour, is banned in Australia and most European countries.

Another common food additive, MSG, found in canned soups and vegetables and processed meats, is known to cause changes in blood pressure, irregular heartbeat, and diarrhea, among others ailments. It can also cause weight gain.

Labeling laws help us make informed choices. Read food labels carefully.

# Genetically Modified Organisms

GMO, genetically modified organism, is a label given to the process of taking genes, bacteria, or viruses from one species and inserting them into another to create plants that have not evolved naturally or to create species that have never reproduced in nature. It is a different process from the common process of cross-pollination, tissue culture, or crossbreeding two plants of different species or varieties, usually from closely or distantly related individuals. GMOs may take only one gene of a plant to inoculate into another or inoculate bacteria or viruses to into plant cells to change the makeup of the new plant.

# How GMOs Are Created

Plants are genetically modified four ways. Here is a simplified explanation of each process.

- Biolistic: Known as ballistic bombardment, heavy metal particles such as gold or tungsten are coated with a gene to be adopted by the plant and then fired with gunpowder into a plant cell.
- Agrobacterium: The DNA of this type of bacteria is transferred to create tumors in plants into which genes can be cut from and pasted into.
- Electroporation: Electricity is used to create pores through which genes can be taken up and incorporated into plant gnomes.
- Gene knockout: A process that knocks out a gene in a plant that is undesirable or inhibits the function of a new gene that will be introduced.

Regardless of which foreign gene, bacteria, or virus is inserted into a plant, the process of insertion, followed by the cloning of that cell into a plant, causes collateral damage to the plant's natural DNA. There can be thousands of mutations throughout the DNA that can create both intended and unintended results. As an intended result of genetic modification, for example, the level of omega-3 fatty acids can be increased. However, the unexpected mutations can also introduce new allergens or toxins, or elevate levels of existing harmful proteins. Neither the companies that create the GMOs, nor federal regulators screen for most of these types of unexpected side effects.

The six most commonly genetically modified (GM) food crops being grown for commercial uses are soy, corn, cotton (used for cooking oils), canola (used for cooking oils), sugar beets (used for sugar production), and alfalfa (used for animal feed). All six are engineered to be herbicide tolerant, meaning they can be sprayed with herbicides like Roundup without being killed. Only the weeds around the crops are destroyed. Some corn and cotton varieties are altered to produce their own toxic insecticides from within, so when an insect eats the corn or cotton plant, the bug's stomach ruptures.

Other less common GM plants are Hawaiian papaya, varieties of crookneck squash, and a small amount of zucchini. GM ingredients are in an estimated 70% or more of all processed foods. The *Huffington Post* includes milk as a GMO product as well because of the recombinant bovine growth hormone given to cows to improve their milk production, which is passed on to us when we consume their milk or milk products.

## The Controversy Around GMOs

There are many controversies surrounding the use of foods and other products derived from genetically modified crops. The areas of dispute are:

- Labeling of GM foods
- Role of government regulators
- Objectivity of scientific research and publication
- Impact of GM crops on health and the environment
- Effect on pesticide resistance
- Impact of such crops for farmers
- Role of the crops in feeding the world population

There are major health and advocacy organizations that are both for and against the use of GMOs in food production. Those who support the use of GM foods are the American Association for the Advancement of Science, the American Medical Association, the National Academies of Science, and the Royal Society of Medicine. These proponents believe the use of GM seeds increases food production for the growing world's population. They further believe the GM foods pose no greater risk to human health than conventional food.

The groups who oppose the use of GM foods include the Organic Consumers Association, the Union of Concerned

Scientists, Greenpeace, Friends of the Earth, GMWatch, Institute for Responsible Technology, and the Institute of Science in Society. These organizations do not believe the risks have been adequately identified and managed, and that the long-term effect of the GM food on humans has not been determined. They are also concerned about the concentration of seeds in the hands of a limited number of multinational corporations.

# GMO Seeds and the Consolidation of the Food Supply

Consolidation of the food supply among several major corporations is a serious concern. As of 2011, 10 companies control 73% of the seed market throughout the world. United States corporations control approximately 50% of the global seeds. Monsanto controls the biggest share of seeds (27%), followed by DuPont (17%) and Land O'Lakes (4%). European companies control the remaining seeds.

Due to end-user agreements that limit what can be done with the seeds, research on GM plants or seeds has been constrained. Because there are proprietary issues, seeds are not available to most scientists. The *Scientific American*, in August 2009, as reported by Wikipedia, noted that several studies initially approved by seed companies were later blocked from publication when they returned "unflattering" results.

# Federal Policy

The criteria used by the federal government to determine if a GM food is safe is whether or not the food is *substantially equivalent* to non-genetically engineered foods that are already accepted to be fit for human consumption. Critics of the *substantially equivalent* criteria say it is vague, not scientifically sound, and limits the amount of research that can be required to determine if the food is safe. Because of the many restrictions placed on long-term research for the safety of

GM foods, there is little conclusive evidence of its effects on humans. The US does not require GM foods to be labeled so consumers can identify the products. The opponents to GM foods propose either a mandatory labeling or a moratorium on such products.

**Federal Drug Administration policy.** FDA policy developed in 1992 states:

> The agency is not aware of any information showing that foods derived by these new methods differ from other foods in a meaningful or uniform way, or that, as a class, foods developed by the new techniques present any different or greater safety concern that foods developed by traditional plant breeding.

Therefore, the FDA claims that no safety studies are needed.

Thousands of memos made public after 1992 indicated a very different story. FDA scientists were very aware of and warned of possible allergies, toxins, and new diseases created by the GM products. They urged the agency to conduct long-term studies. The FDA ignored their scientists. As is the case with other federal agencies, there is a close relationship between senior staff of the regulatory agencies and the entities for which they have oversight. Because the federal government does not oversee the regulation of GM food products, the oversight for food safety now falls to the agencies that develop the GM food products. In the case of GM foods, the major US corporations that produce them, Monsanto, DuPont (Pioneer), and Land O'Lakes, would be responsible for insuring their safety.

**Labeling or banning GM food products.** Sixty-seven countries, including France, Italy, Germany, Spain, the United Kingdom, Portugal, Russia, Switzerland, Norway, Australia, New Zealand, Thailand, the Philippines, Saudi Arabia, Egypt, Brazil, and Paraguay, have banned the use of some genetically engineered food/crops or require mandatory labeling.

Various states within the United States have attempted to mandate labeling of GM foods and/or ban the production of GM crops.

Legislation is under discussion or pending in 20 states. Opponents of the legislation have contributed billions of dollars to defeat the new measures or laws. Monsanto alone contributed more than $6 billion in the 2013 lobbying efforts against the labeling of GM products. Other sponsors against labeling include PepsiCo, Coca-Cola, General Mills, and Nestlé.

## GMOs, Allergies, Leaky Gut, and Cancer

According to the Centers for Disease Control and Prevention statistics, hospital-confirmed extreme food allergies have been steadily increasing over the past 15 years. Soy allergies increased by 50% after the introduction of GM soy in the UK. Natural soy does not contain the allergen. GM corn also contains allergens not found in natural corn. When someone is allergic to one substance in their food they can become more susceptible to reactions from other substances in other foods. If GM proteins trigger an allergen reaction, the danger is compounded by the fact the new genes can transfer into the DNA of human gut bacteria. They may continuously produce the protein allergen within our intestines, worsening the original allergic reaction and creating others. These conditions place an enormous load on our immune systems.

**GMOs and leaky gut.** Based on animal feeding studies, case studies, and the properties of these crops, GMOs are believed to increase incidences of celiac disease and gluten sensitivity, disorders that have more than doubled in the last two decades. A significant percentage of patients diagnosed with celiac disease and gluten sensitivity have leaky gut. In leaky gut the junctures between cells lining the intestinal wall open up, allowing the contents of the intestines to enter the bloodstream before they are fully digested. Food particles, food proteins, toxins, and gut bacteria entering the bloodstream cause an inflammatory reaction and lead to a wide range of autoimmune conditions and diseases.

**GMOs and Bt toxins.** There is a strong correlation between the rise of Bt corn in the US diet and incidences of gastrointestinal disorders, including leaky gut. Bt corn has a built-in pesticide from a gene from soil bacteria called Bacillus thuringiensis, or Bt, and the corn may be highly toxic.

Bt corn, designed to destroy the stomachs of insects, may also do the same to our guts. Several peer-reviewed studies have shown Bt toxins from the GM corn are not inert on human cells, as purported by manufacturers, but can be toxic. In high concentrations, the toxins can disrupt the intestinal membranes, causing the fluid to leak out, hence leaky gut. The authors compare the process to what happens to the bugs when they ingest Bt corn. Anecdotal evidence brings home this supposition. As the acreage of Bt corn has increased, there has been a corresponding increase in the diagnosis of inflammatory bowel disease, peritonitis, constipation, and deaths due to intestinal infection in humans. Deaths due to intestinal infections went from 100,000 to 350,000 in the span of 13 years, beginning about 6 years after the introduction of Bt corn. The deaths increased as the acres of Bt corn increased.

Further, a 2011 Canadian study discovered that 93% of the pregnant women tested had Bt toxin from genetically modified corn in their blood. Eighty percent of their unborn fetuses did too. The Bt toxins were believed to come from the meat and dairy products from corn-fed animals. The authors concluded that the Bt toxin remains intact during the digestive process of the animals and is passed on to the human digestive system.

**GM food products and cancer in rats.** An article published in the journal *Food and Chemical Toxicity* reported the results of a study that implicated the consumption of GM foods in cancer in rats. For two years rats in the study were given either Roundup-tolerant GM maize, cultivated either with or without Roundup, and Roundup alone, at levels permitted in drinking water and GM crops in the United States. The rats developed many more tumors and died earlier than the controls. The rats also developed tumors when glyphosate (Roundup) was added to their drinking water. The results of the research paper were highly controversial and the authors were forced to withdraw their paper when a former Monsanto employee became associate editor of the journal. The associate editor stated there was no relationship between the two events. The authors stand by their work.

# Insecticides, Fertilizers, and the Environment

It takes approximately 1,000 years to produce 2.5 inches of fertile soil. Ideally, that soil contains microorganisms, fungi, beneficial species of bacteria, beneficial nematodes, microarthropods, and earthworms. These organisms take the mineral material in the soil and convert it into materials plants use for growth. Chemical fertilizers disrupt this process and may be poisoning the soil. One application of Roundup may irreversibly change the microorganisms in the soil. Genetically modified crops initially increase crop yield, but over time, the yield drops. Crop growers need to increase their use of fertilizer to maintain their yields, continuously changing the composition of and life within the soil.

In the early 70s, Monsanto developed, patented, and marketed the glyphosate molecule, the primary ingredient in its herbicide, Roundup. It is estimated that nearly one billion pounds of glyphosate are sprayed on our crops each year. Recent research reported on the GreenMedInfo website found that extremely small concentrations of glyphosate, 450 times lower than used in agricultural application, induced DNA damage in human cells.

Glyphosate is contaminating our water and air. As a result of runoff, it is contaminating ground water stored in our natural subterranean aquifers, a critical water source for generations. It is also present in the air. One 2011 study found glyphosate in 60 to 100% of all US air and rain samples in the regions where glyphosate was applied.

A new kidney disease (chronic kidney disease of unknown etiology/CKDu) has been linked to glyphosate use. When powdered glyphosate is mixed with water that contains high amounts of calcium, magnesium, strontium, and iron (commonly known as hard water), it creates a mixture that is toxic to kidneys. Researchers are able to track the origins of the CKDu by noting geographically where the fertilizer containing glyphosate is used.

## The Controversy Continues

In spite of the accumulating evidence, the GMOs continue to cause controversy. An international group of more than 90 scientists, academics, and physicians released a statement in October 2013 stating there is "no scientific consensus" on the safety of GM foods and crops. It was a rebuttal to claims from the GM industry that there "is scientific consensus" that genetically modified organisms are generally found safe for human and animal consumption. Long-term studies on the effect of GM products on human health are needed to validate or repudiate these opposing points of view. Companies that produce GMOs need to make their seeds available to determine their long-term effects on human and animal health.

## We're Beginning to Make Better Food Choices

Fast foods and processed foods are probably going to be with us forever. We love their flavors and their convenience. But we need to make more healthy choices and there are indications we're making progress. Public awareness and new labeling laws are having an effect on our eating habits. Sales of organic products have climbed from $3.6 billion to $24.4 billion in the last ten years. First quarter earnings from McDonald's (April 2014) are down 2.7% to $1.24 billion compared to the first quarter of 2013. Eighteen states experienced a decline in obesity rates among preschool children from low-income families after a comprehensive approach to obesity prevention was adopted. Hopefully, the same will be true soon for adult obesity. What is evident is the *rate of increase* for obesity is slowing for adults.

Campaigns to label genetically modified foods are spreading across the nation. Lacking federal government leadership, the states have taken the initiative. In spite of the food industry's millions of dollars and misleading advertisements, California and Washington ballot measures to mandate GMO labeling were only narrowly defeated, 51% to 49%. GMO labeling will be on the ballot in Oregon in November 2014. Vermont passed the first unconditional statewide labeling law for genetically engineered foods in May 2014. The Grocers Association and three other trade associations have filed a lawsuit in federal court to block the new law, but it is being vigorously defended by the citizens of Vermont. It's a people's movement, and although it may take time, people want to know what they are eating so they can make informed choices.

CHAPTER 3

# Pills for Profit

M Y FRIEND ROSE WAS DIAGNOSED WITH CHRONIC MYELOID
leukemia (CLM) in 2008. The life expectancy, depending on
the stage of the disease, is between five and ten years. Fortunately
for Rose, a drug sold by the pharmaceutical company Novartis,
Gleevec, is in a way a miracle drug. Introduced in 2001, Gleevec has
dramatically increased the survival rate and changed CLM from a
fatal disease to a chronic, manageable one. As long as Rose takes the
drug, she should lead a normal life for many years. The down side to
this drug is its cost: $7,800 for a thirty-day supply.

Millions of people are alive today because of lifesaving drugs.
Polio, tuberculosis, and malaria have been virtually wiped out. Antibiotics have prevented millions from dying from infections. Cancer
drugs, drugs to reduce blood pressure, and drugs to manage heart
disease, diabetes, and autoimmune diseases have prolonged millions
of lives. The list goes on, but there is a dark side to this boon to
mankind—and it's money.

The United States drug industry is the second most profitable
business in the country, second only to the gas and oil industry.
Developing and selling prescriptions has become a billion (billion with a b) dollar industry. Many lifesaving cancer drugs, like
Gleevec, are priced so high that without medical insurance and/
or patient assistance giveaways, people would be unable to use the
medication. Unfortunately, nearly one in five patients cannot afford

them and aren't eligible for assistance. Without the drug, they will die. Gleevec earned Novartis $4.7 billion dollars last year. Between 2001 and 2012 the top ten drug companies earned $711 billion dollars. In 2012 eleven of the twelve cancer drugs the Food and Drug Administration approved were priced at more than $100,000 per year, double the average annual household income.

A study done by the group Families USA reported that American's major drug companies' profits far exceeded their cost for research and development. The drug companies are spending more than twice as much on marketing, advertising, and administration than they do on research and development. Here is an example of their net profits over the past nine years.

### Net Profits for the Top 11 Global Pharmaceutical Companies, 2003–2012. (In billions of US dollars)

| | |
|---|---|
| Johnson & Johnson | $105.8 |
| Pfizer | $100.4 |
| Novartis | $83.1 |
| GlaxoSmithKline | $77.8 |
| Roche | $73.3 |
| Merck | $59.1 |
| AstraZeneca | $58.9 |
| Sanofi-Aventis | $57.7 |
| Abbott Laboratories | $40.6 |
| Eli Lilly | $27.7 |
| Bristol-Myers Squibb | $27.0 |

# How Did Drug Companies Become So Profitable?

Recently, a group of more than 120 cancer researchers and doctors published a paper in the American Society of Hematology's medical journal, *Blood*, calling the prices of cancer drugs exorbitant and unjustifiable. When Gleevec was first introduced in 2001, the annual cost was $30,000. That price has more than doubled over the years and now wholesales for $76,000 per year. Dr. Hagop Kantarjian, the lead author of the paper, told CNNMoney reporter Stacy Crowley, "These price increases do not reflect the cost of development of drugs or the benefit they provide to the patient. They are simply related to the drug companies' wish to increase profits beyond a reasonable range." Top-tier cancer drugs cost twice as much in the United States as they do in parts of Europe, China, Canada, and the United Kingdom, where the governments set a limit on pricing.

Many drugs related to lifestyle diseases, such as heart disease, obesity, diabetes, and autoimmune diseases, are also exorbitantly priced. In spite of the huge cost, physicians have come to rely on medication more often than the cost effective, and in many cases more healthful, diet and lifestyle changes to address the needs of their patients. There are several reasons for this. Very few hours of medical training, including coursework and internships, are dedicated to nutrition and/or the benefits of exercise. Once doctors are in practice, the brief office visits do not leave time to address these kinds of interventions, nor is follow-up time allotted for or funded by the insurance companies. Continuing education during the doctors' years of practice often comes from drug company representatives or respected members of their own professions who are paid by the pharmaceutical companies.

Patients bear a responsibility too. Pervasive television and print media sponsored by the drug companies urge consumers to ask their doctors to prescribe the companies' drugs, whose benefits seem to be life-changing, ignoring the long list of adverse side effects. Medications are an easier fix than lifestyle and diet changes, and patients often request drugs they have identified from advertisements. As a result, drugs are often seen by the patient and the doctor alike as the most expedient and efficient way to provide care. Our healthcare system is a disease system, designed to react to symptoms and disease, associating treatment with medications rather than diet and lifestyle changes. Unfortunately, this practice supports the pharmaceuticals, and as they've grown and prospered, illegal actions and practices have come to light.

The interconnectedness of drug companies and their paid representatives is so widespread that it is difficult to tell fact from fiction. Dr. Peter C. Gøtzsche, author of *Deadly Medicines and Organised Crime: How Big Pharma Has Corrupted Healthcare,* notes that US drug companies have more than three times as many law violations as other American companies—adjusting for company size. Charges include international bribery and corruption, and criminal negligence in the unsafe manufacture of drugs. He says:

> Almost every type of person who can affect the interests of the industry has been bribed: doctors, hospital administrators, cabinet ministers, health inspectors, customs officers, tax assessors, drug registration officials, factory inspectors, pricing officials and political parties. (p. 39)

Richard Smith, MD, former editor of the prestigious *British Medical Journal,* wrote one of the introductions to Peter Gøtzsche's book. Smith says:

> Laws that are requiring companies to declare payments to doctors are showing a very high proportion of doctors are beholden to the drug industry and that many are being paid six figure sums for advising companies or giving talks on their behalf. It's hard to escape the conclusion that these "key opinion leaders" are being bought. They are the "hired guns" of the industry. (p. viii)

## The Human Cost of Drugs

Drugs save millions of lives each year, but they can be dangerous. Drug-related deaths are the third largest cause of death, behind heart disease and cancer. Dr. Gøtzsche summarizes the probable numbers of deaths caused by bad drugs. (p. 260) Here are two examples:

- By 2004 rofecoxib (used to treat arthritis and other conditions causing chronic or acute pain) had likely caused about 1,200,000 deaths worldwide because of thrombosis before it was withdrawn.
- By 2007 olanzapine (used to treat schizophrenia and acute manic episodes associated with bipolar I disorder) had likely killed about 200,000 people worldwide.

An estimated 450,000 preventable medication-related adverse events occur in the US every year.

## The Cost of Doing Business

The drug companies have often misled the public on the safety and efficacy of their products. In a rush to get them to pharmacy shelves, drugs are often advertised and sold before all their side effects are known over time, or they may be marketed for conditions for which they were not tested. Merck's Vioxx, an anti-inflammatory drug used to relieve signs and symptoms of arthritis, acute pain in adults, and painful menstrual cycles, is an example of the problem. It alone killed more than 60,000 people before it was withdrawn from the market.

The legal settlement, which required Merck to withdraw Vioxx from the marketplace, required Merck to pay $58 million in restitution to states. It is the largest monetary settlement that a group of states has obtained in a pharmaceutical advertising case. The settlement funds pay for attorneys' fees, future enforcement, and consumer education. The settlement places restrictions on Merck's future conduct, including:

- Prohibits the use of deceptive scientific data when marketing new drugs to doctors.

- Prohibits Merck from "ghost writing" articles and studies for publication.
- Requires disclosure of conflicts of interest when Merck's promotional speakers make presentations at supposedly independent Continuing Medical Education programs.
- Requires Merck to submit clinical trial results of FDA-approved Merck products to the National Library of Medicine.

The federal government has also prosecuted other pharmaceutical companies for similar practices. Recent findings by the US government declared that Pfizer, another major drug company, was officially guilty of violating the RICO (racketeering influenced corrupt organization) Act for fraudulent marketing of the epilepsy drug Neurontin. The company was fined $142 million. Pfizer marketed the drug as appropriate for several disorders, including neuropathic pain and migraines, even though the claims were unsupported by scientific evidence. Pfizer was also fined $2.3 billion in 2009 for illegally promoting off-label uses for four of its drugs.

The largest financial settlement for fraudulent activities to date was $3 billion paid by GlaxoSmithKline (GSK) for the inappropriate sales and marketing practices of several of its drugs, including Avandia, a drug for diabetes, and Paxil and Wellbutrin, drugs for combating depression. Between 1999 and 2007, Avandia is estimated to have caused over 80,000 heart attacks. Paxil was unlawfully marketed to children and adolescents for depression, although the drug was approved only for adults. Wellbutrin was marketed for weight loss and sexual dysfunction.

GSK announced in December 2012 that it would no longer pay medical professionals and physicians to represent and educate their peers about the manufactures' drugs. GSK also stopped paying its sales representatives based on the number of prescriptions that doctors wrote. Both were conditions of the US Department of Justice 2011 settlement.

Dr. Gøtzsche, in preparing his manuscript for *Deadly Medicines and Organised Crime: How Big Pharma Has Corrupted Healthcare,* investigated the illegal behavior of pharmaceutical manufacturers by conducting a Google search combining the names of the 10 largest drug companies and the word "fraud." He found hundreds of violations. In his book he lists those companies that were convicted of criminal offenses between 2007 and 2012 and the amount of the fines or settlements they were ordered to pay. The most common criminal offenses included illegal marketing, recommending drugs for off-label uses, misrepresentation of research results, hiding data on harmful effects, and Medicaid and Medicare fraud. The top fines were: GlaxoSmithKline, $3 billion in 2011; Pfizer, $2.3 billion in 2009; and Abbott, $1.5 billion in 2012. The other seven companies' fines ranged from 1.4 billion to $423 million.

The huge fines imposed on the leading drug companies do not seem to deter their efforts to improve their profit margins. The fines are simply the cost of doing business.

# The Federal Drug Administration

The role of the Federal Drug Administration (FDA) is to regulate almost every facet of prescription drugs, including testing, manufacturing, labeling, advertising, marketing, efficacy, and safety. In 1992 Congress passed the Prescription Drug User Fee Act, which allows the drug companies to pay the FDA for its services, putting the fox in the chicken house and making the scientists at the FDA susceptible to pressure from the companies. Research documents this predictable scenario. A poll showed that 61% of FDA scientists are aware of political interference in the approval process. Seventy percent of the FDA scientists are not confident products approved by the FDA are safe. Sixty percent lack confidence in the FDA's safety monitoring of marketed drugs.

The practices and ethics of the pharmaceutical companies in the research and development process of new drugs have been called into question. Drummond Rennie, Deputy Director of *The Journal of the American Medical Association*, also wrote in the introduction to Gøtzsche's book:

> There already exist hundreds of reports of scientific studies, and many books written, about the way pharmaceutical companies pervert the scientific process and, using this massive wealth, all too often work against the patients they claim to help. (p. x)

Among those Rennie mentioned is Marcia Angell, a former editor of the *New England Journal of Medicine* and author of *The Truth About the Drug Companies: How They Deceive Us and What To Do About It* (2005).

## An Alternative Point of View

Marcia Angell has her critics. On the other side of the pills for profit issue, John LaMattina, a contributor to *Forbes* online who covers drug research and development in the pharmaceutical industry, disputes claims regarding attacks on the big drug companies, calling into question the information in Dr. Angell's book. He notes that the FDA reported, "Much like 2011, 2012 has proven a great year for patients, with the approval of 35 innovative drugs." Many of the new drugs come from small biotech companies, but LaMattina also defends Pfizer and Merck for new drug approvals and notes that "many of the new drugs have been developed through innovative paradigms and experimental methods developed by scientists and physicians in the pharmaceutical industry." He also takes to task accusations that medical experts are being paid off by pharmaceutical companies to influence national health guidelines to favor the greater use of drugs. He uses cholesterol-lowering drugs as an example of good medical science that has reduced heart attacks and strokes.

# Pharmaceutical-Induced Nutritional Deficiencies

Nutritional deficiencies caused by the drugs are seldom taken into consideration when medical professionals prescribe pharmaceuticals. Statins, for example, may deplete or interfere with the activity of Coenzyme Q10, beta-carotene, vitamins B3 and B12, vitamins E, K, and D, zinc, magnesium, calcium, folic acid, and phosphorus. Colesevelam (Welchol), used to treat elevated cholesterol, may interfere with or deplete similar vitamins, including the mineral iron. Ciprofloxacin (Cipro, Ciloxan), an antibacterial agent, may increase the need for or deplete biotin, inositol, thiamin, riboflavin, niacin, vitamins B6, B12, and K, and zinc, along with the probiotics Bifidobacteria bifidum and Lactobacillus acidophilus. Glyburide plus Metformin (Glucovance), used to treat diabetes, may reduce the body's supply of folic acid, vitamin B12, sodium, and Coenzyme Q10.

Other popular prescription drugs that deplete nutrients are prednisone (Deltasone, Liquid Pred) used to treat inflammatory ailments of the skin, gastrointestinal tract, and other areas of the body. The nutrients depleted or interfered with include vitamins A, B6, C, D, and K, and folic acid, calcium, magnesium, potassium, selenium, and zinc. Ranitidine (Zantac), used for ailments related to digestive organs or processes, may deplete or interfere with the functioning of thiamin, folic acid, calcium, iron, zinc, and vitamins B12 and D. These examples are a sampling of the effects of various pharmaceuticals that, in addition to the other side effects, can cause unsuspected conditions that can weaken the body.

# A Statin in Every Medicine Cabinet

A perfect example of the pervasiveness of the prescription drug culture is the new 2012 guidelines for the use of statins, a cholesterol-lowering drug. The guidelines introduced by experts from the American Heart Association and the American College of

Cardiology will greatly increase the number of Americans taking statins. Rather than wait until a certain level of cholesterol is reached, patients are advised to take a statin drug if they already have a heart disease, if their LDL cholesterol is 190 or more, if they're middle-aged with type 2 diabetes, if they are at risk for a stroke, or if they're between the ages of 40 and 75 years of age with an estimated 10-year risk of heart disease. The committee recommended that doctors should use known risks for cardiovascular disease, including age, cholesterol levels, blood pressure, smoking, and diabetes in prescribing the drugs. The committee also suggested that about one-third of adults at risk for a heart attack or stroke who had not been diagnosed could benefit from statins. The guidelines do include recommendations for lifestyle changes, such as brisk walking for about 40 minutes three or four times a week.

Critics of the new policy are speaking out. Authors Sultan and Hynes, in an article titled "The Ugly Side of Statins, Systemic Appraisal of the Contemporary Un-Known Unknowns," published in the *Open Journal of Endocrine and Metabolic Disease*, did a comprehensive review of PubMed, EM-BASE, and Cochrane Review databases of articles relating to cardiovascular primary prevention and regenerative programs. The article abstract states:

> Not only is there a dearth of evidence for primary cardiovascular protection, there is ample evidence to show that statins actually augment cardiovascular risk in women, patients with Diabetes Mellitus and in the young. Furthermore statins are associated with triple the risk of coronary artery and aortic artery calcification.

The recommendations for increasing the use of statins will be a boon for the drug companies. Lipitor, a commonly prescribed medication for lowering cholesterol, costs an average $100 per month in the US. It is an example of over-pricing to increase the profit margin. In New Zealand, a prescription for Lipitor is $6. In South Africa it is $11, and in Spain, $13. With one-half of the adults in the US between the ages of 40 and 75 years of age on some form of cholesterol-lowering medication, the profits for the pharmaceuticals will be astronomical. The absolute irony is that there is little scientific evidence that the medication will have the benefits projected by the new guidelines.

## What If We All Went Walking?

Authors Naci and Loannidis, in a meta-analysis of 305 randomized control trials with 339,274 participants, found:

> Exercise and many drug interventions are often potentially similar in terms of their mortality benefits in the secondary prevention of coronary heart disease, rehabilitation after stroke, treatment of heart failure and prevention of diabetes. (p. 1)

Predictably, the amount of evidence on the lifesaving benefits of exercise is considerably smaller than the evidence on drug interventions. There are few exercise and drug studies comparing the effectiveness and outcomes of each. The authors note that in the body of scientific research studies, drug trials far outweigh those that involved exercise (57 exercise trials out of 305 trials), and fewer people participated (14,716 participants in trials that involved exercise out of 339,274 participants), noting the bias that exists against exercise interventions that could yield better results and more durable gains, and without the side effects that come with many drugs.

Naci and Loannidis use as an example the change in clinical practice guidelines in the US for the use of statin drugs. Earlier versions of the national cholesterol education program guidelines advised the use of statins only after exhausting interventions for intensive lifestyle changes for the prevention of coronary heart disease in people with high cholesterol. The threshold for prescribing statins has progressively lowered until the latest recommendations for prescribing statins include almost 50% of the population of the country.

Naci and Loannidis recommend more funding for drug and

exercise comparisons. Given the limited amount of funding available, regulators should consider requiring pharmaceutical sponsors of new drugs to include exercise intervention comparisons as a component of drug trials. The following is an example of what might become commonplace.

In a trial with 156 patients with major depression, the outcome was similar for those who were randomly selected to do an exercise program and those who received sertraline (Zoloft). However, six months later, only 30% of the exercise group was depressed as compared with 52% of the group who took the drug. The Cochrane Database Systematic Review also reported similar findings. Drugs were no more effective than exercise and the effect of exercise was more durable. It is also cheaper with fewer negative side effects.

One of the reasons there are few studies comparing exercise and drug interventions is that such studies would discourage drug use as the first intervention, rather than the last, and would dramatically cut into the revenues of the pharmaceutical companies and their supporters. Drugs can be a great blessing, but also a curse. Many health practitioners, particularly alternative providers, do recommend diet and lifestyle changes before introducing drug therapy, or in close collaboration with drug therapy. It is up to you to choose your healthcare providers and the drugs they prescribe with care.

SECTION TWO

# How Things Work

CHAPTER 4

# Why Your Brain Needs Good Food

Your brain needs nutritious food to maintain its 100 billion nerve cells and 200 billion supporting cells. It's composed of protein and fat and fueled by carbohydrates.

Although the brain weighs only three pounds, it takes a disproportionate amount of fuel and energy to function. When you eat a meal, the food is converted to brain cells through digestion. During the digestive process, proteins become amino acids, fats become fatty acids, and carbohydrates become glucose and glycogen. Amino acids provide structure for cells and produce hormones. Fatty acids are used for insulation, to make cholesterol, and for fuel if there is a shortage of glucose. Glucose and glycogen are sources of fuel. The brain has one of the richest networks of blood vessels in the body. Your brain uses 25% of the oxygen you breathe. It is also highly susceptible to toxins and inflammation. The brain is both dynamic and delicate.

## The Inner Workings of the Brain

The brain is one of the most complicated and miraculous things on Earth. It's the master computer of the body, directing the mind and managing the body. It does so by sending electrochemical messages from one neuron to another, creating a network that directs thoughts, actions, feelings, and bodily functions. As the trillions of nerve cells communicate and interact, we are able to experience ourselves as conscious human beings.

The neurons, or nerve cells, are the workhorses of the brain. The glial cells (neuroglia) support the neurons. The glial cells regulate the environment of the brain by providing structure, nutritional support, insulation, and protection from pathogens. There are about three glial cells to one neuron.

Throughout the brain, all communication occurs via the nerve cells. Each type of neuron, made up of proteins, DNA, and other molecules, has its own set of genes that determines its function. Myelin, a coating made up of seventy percent fat, surrounds many of the neurons. Some nerve cells are very long, from the top of the head to the toes; others are fractions of an inch. Each nerve cell sends out axons that carry messages from the cell body. Extending from the axons are smaller dendrite branches. The dendrites receive messages from other axons. The messages pass between them at gaps called synapses. Receptors at the synapse receive the messages and they're passed along the nerve cells by an electrochemical charge. The cell bodies, which are held in place by fatty acids, have openings. When the messages enter the cell bodies through these openings, nerve impulses occur, cocktails of chemicals are released, and the messages are delivered. The messages, neurotransmitters, are made up of proteins and amino acids and create the electrical impulse. There are trillions of synapses on trillions of nerve cells that receive the neurotransmitters. Each nerve cell may have up to 10,000 synapses.

The neurotransmitters have particular shapes that fit into matching receptor molecules. When the neurotransmitters attach to their receptor molecules, they stimulate the molecule to perform its unique action. A healthy, well-functioning neuron can be directly linked to tens of thousands of other neurons, creating a totality of more than a hundred trillion connections that are each capable of performing 200 calculations per second.

The complexity of the human brain is astounding. Neuroscientists analyzed a section of a mouse brain that was the volume of $\frac{1}{100,000}$ the size of a grain of salt. Within that miniscule section of brain matter, they found a thousand axons and about 80 dendrites, each making about 600 connections. The human brain is 3,000 times larger than a mouse brain.

# Hormones and Brain Functioning

Normal hormone levels are necessary for neurotransmitter functioning and brain health. Balanced hormones facilitate neuron branching and plasticity to create new neurons and synapses, and to manage neural pathways and neural processes. Nutritious food is crucial for developing healthy hormones. The following four hormones are most critical for neurotransmitter functioning.

**Acetylcholine.** Acetylcholine is a major neurotransmitter, active in the hippocampus, important for conversion of short-term memory to long-term memory. Blood sugar imbalances and processed vegetable fats interfere with acetylcholine function. Symptoms of acetylcholine impairment are the same symptoms as Alzheimer's. Natural fats, avocados, nuts, olive oil, and animal fats, particularly those from pasture-raised animals, are beneficial to acetylcholine production.

**Serotonin.** Serotonin is a neurotransmitter found in blood platelets and serum. Serotonin is manufactured in the midbrain and is dependent on adequate light for production. Low levels of serotonin are associated with anger and aggressiveness, irritable bowel syndrome, fibromyalgia, and various brain disorders, including depression, anxiety disorders, and obsessive-compulsive disorder. Excessive serotonin is linked to debilitating shyness, nervousness, feeling vulnerable to criticism, and fear of not being liked. Serotonin is converted into melatonin in the brain's pineal gland and can affect sleep patterns. The production of serotonin is dependent on sufficient levels of iron and amino acids.

**GABA.** GABA (gamma-aminobutyric acid) is a neurotransmitter associated with anxiety and nervousness. GABA is so critical for brain health that it is produced in all neurons. Hypoglycemia, insulin resistance, and diabetes disturb glucose production and, therefore, GABA production. Stress, lifestyle issues, toxic chemicals, gluten intolerance, celiac disease, and autoimmune diseases also affect GABA functioning. GABA is produced when glucose is metabolized for energy. Fruits and vegetables and whole grains are good sources of glucose.

**Dopamine.** Dopamine is the feel good hormone that enables us to focus, to be motivated, to feel good about ourselves, and to feel pleasure. Dopamine is necessary for frontal lobe functioning that regulates mood, attention, learning, libido, and motor coordination. People with low dopamine levels may experience depression, lack of motivation, hopelessness, feelings of worthlessness, inability to concentrate, inability to handle stress, irritability, and self-destructive thoughts. Excessive levels of dopamine are associated with psychosis, schizophrenia, hyperactivity, and high libido. Overall brain health, stress, and poor blood sugar regulation are contributors to dopamine imbalances. Many antipsychotic medications target dopamine receptors. Adequate amounts of protein and fat, coupled with a limited amount of carbohydrates promote dopamine production.

**Other important hormones.** Estrogen, progesterone, and testosterone all impact acetylcholine, serotonin, GABA, and dopamine performance. The thyroid gland is also connected to the four hormones and contributes to brain function. A healthy thyroid facilitates good synapsis connections, dampens brain inflammation, and promotes healthy neurotransmitter functioning. Foods rich in iodine, such as eggs, fish, and sea vegetables, support thyroid function. A balanced, nutrient rich diet of carbohydrates, protein, and fat promote the function of all hormones.

# Brain Diseases and Disorders

The number of people with brain diseases and disorders is on the increase. In 2010, 3.8 million people, or 15% of people age 71 or older, had dementia. Scientists forecast numbers of persons with dementia will increase to 9.1 million by 2040. Twenty-two percent, or about 5.4 million people age 71 and older, now have mild cognitive impairment. About 12% of those people will develop Alzheimer's each year.

When something goes wrong in the brain, speech, muscular coordination, logical thought, and memories may be lost. As we age, we lose some ability to quickly recall names or nouns, or forget where we left our keys. This is the normal process of aging. Dementia or cognitive decline may be developing if our ability to think and remember major events declines substantially. Unfortunately, as the number of people with extended lifespans has increased, so has the number of people with dementia.

**Dementia.** Dementia is a common name for various diseases and conditions that damage brain cells. It accounts for the loss of mental functions, such as thinking, memory, and reasoning, that is severe enough to interfere with a person's daily activities. Alzheimer's disease accounts for 50 to 60% of dementia cases. The risk factors for dementia and Alzheimer's disease are similar to the risk factors for other common Western diseases, such as cardiovascular disease, glucose intolerance, insulin resistance, type 2 diabetes, hypertension, and obesity. Stroke, toxic reactions to excessive alcohol or drug use, infections of the brain or spinal cord, and head injuries also cause dementia.

**Alzheimer's disease.** Alzheimer's disease is the most common form of dementia. The cause of Alzheimer's disease is unclear. Some researchers believe the tangles and plaques that are characteristic of the disease are caused by the gradual accumulation of abnormal protein deposits. Others believe the cause to be a misfiring of brain neurons, general inflammation, or genetic malfunction. Inflammation and oxidation contribute to Alzheimer's, just as they do for heart disease, diabetes, cancer, and aging itself.

Symptoms of Alzheimer's begin with forgetfulness and mild confusion. As the disease progresses, thinking and reasoning become difficult, judgment and decision-making are impaired, the ability to perform familiar tasks declines, and changes in personality and behavior occur. As more cells die, the brain shrinks in size, and the symptoms become more severe. The ultimate result is death. The disease manifests in different ways with each person. As of 2012, more than 1,000 clinical trials had been or were being conducted to find ways to treat the disease.

**Stroke.** A stroke, or "brain attack" or cerebrovascular accident (CVA), occurs when blood flow is cut off to a part of the brain. If the brain is deprived of blood and oxygen for more than a few seconds, brain cells begin to die. If the stoppage continues, neurological damage, complications, or even death can occur. The symptoms of a stroke include a sudden numbness or weakness of the face, arms, or legs, especially on one side of the body, inability to move one or more limbs on one side of the body, inability to understand or formulate speech, slurred speech, dizziness, lack of coordination, and/or trouble seeing in one or both eyes.

There are two kinds of major strokes, ischemia and hemorrhagic. The ischemia stroke occurs when a blood vessel that supplies blood to the brain is blocked. A hemorrhagic stroke occurs when a blood vessel in the brain becomes weak and bursts, causing blood to leak into the brain. A third kind of stroke, less severe, is a transient ischemic attack (TIA), or mini-stroke. The symptoms generally last less than 24 hours. Up to 40% of all people who experience a TIA will have a major stroke, often within three months.

Epidemiological studies have found that people with one or more of abdominal obesity, high blood pressure, high cholesterol, or insulin resistance are at greater risk for stroke than the general population. Other factors that increase the risks of stoke are smoking, hypertension, and diabetes.

**Atherosclerosis.** The common name for atherosclerosis is hardening of the arteries. It's a disease characterized by the deposit of plaques of fatty material on the inner walls of the arteries. It is the most common underlying cause of heart attacks, heart failure, stroke, and non-Alzheimer's dementia. It appears to be an inflammatory reaction to foreign substances in the blood that causes plaque to form, coating the arteries and constricting blood flow.

## Causes of Brain Deterioration

Our food choices often determine the health of our brains. Chronic inflammation appears to be at the root of most brain diseases and is caused or exacerbated by what we eat. Chronic inflammation destroys neurons and affects brain functioning. Causes of brain inflammation include gut inflammation, oxidation, poor sugar regulation, glycation, and toxins.

**Gut inflammation.** The gut biome acts as a physical barrier to prevent food particles, toxins, yeast, and other disruptions from invading the digestive tract. Small intestinal bacterial overgrowth occurs when the gut biome is compromised. When the good gut flora is gone or disrupted, pathogenic bacteria can populate the gut at will, leading to leaky gut and gut inflammation.

**Oxidation.** Oxidation is a chemical reaction that produces free radicals. Free radicals are a byproduct of the body's metabolism and have many important functions, including helping the immune system fight off disease. However, too many free radicals contribute to tissue damage found in people who experience a stroke and people who have had cancer, schizophrenia, Parkinson's disease, and Alzheimer's disease. While our bodies produce some free radicals, others enter our bodies through the food we eat and through the lungs and skin from the toxins in our environments.

**Poor sugar regulation.** One of the most damaging conditions for the brain is a blood sugar imbalance caused by insulin resistance or diabetes. It has such dire consequences that some researchers refer to Alzheimer's as type 3 diabetes. Glucose is the brain's major fuel source and an even supply of glucose is critical to maintain stable blood sugar levels. When blood sugar levels are unstable, fluctuating rapidly as in insulin resistance and diabetes, brain chemistry, neurotransmitter production, and overall brain function is disrupted.

Insulin resistance is a result of long-term elevated blood sugar levels caused by excess glucose and insulin circulating in the blood. Too much glucose and insulin in the blood causes inflammation. Insulin resistance may progress to diabetes. People with diabetes are twice as likely to succumb to Alzheimer's. Excessive insulin also reduces the brain's ability to clear out amyloid plaques, a brain abnormality that is characteristic of Alzheimer's. It is estimated that one-third of the US population has insulin resistance.

**Glycation and AGEs.** Sugar cooked with protein forms advanced glycosylation end products (AGEs), which produces glycation. Glycation causes oxidation stress and the production of free radicals. Cooking or grilling meats, potatoes, bread, or any other food at temperatures greater than 248 degrees Fahrenheit creates AGEs. AGEs are in the brown crust on anything cooked in the absence of water. All grains, vegetables, fruits, and nuts contain a combination of sugar and protein, which under the right conditions, form AGEs. Food manufacturers add AGEs to foods as flavor enhancers and colorants to improve appearances. Cooking with water, steaming, stewing, or boiling prevents the sugars from binding with the proteins and creating AGEs.

Diets high in AGEs speed up the aging process and the degenerative diseases usually associated with aging. AGE levels are a better indicator of physical or functional age than chronological age. When comparing older subjects (over 60) with younger subjects, scientists have found that AGEs generally increase with age. In the presence of inflammation, oxidative stress, and insulin resistance, AGEs increase regardless of the subject's age.

**Toxins.** In addition to feeding the brain good nutrients, it is important to limit exposure to toxins. As they accumulate in the body, they can damage the brain. We ingest thousands of chemicals from processed food and pesticides and herbicides. We take in more from plastic bottles and food cans. We breathe thousands more in polluted air, from the chemicals used in cleaning and yard maintenance products, and in the manufacturing processes for clothes, furniture, carpets, paints, and other household items.

Lead is a particularly dangerous toxin. Occupational and childhood exposure to lead causes progressive mental decline. What has previously been described as "normal aging" may actually be caused partially by exposure to lead and other toxic metals. Toxins disrupt myelin, the fatty substance around nerves that allows the nerves to carry signals efficiently. When myelin is damaged, a nerve's electrochemical impulse is disrupted and uncoordinated, scrambling or cutting off information being transmitted. Lead also inhibits the action of calcium as a regulator of cell function and disrupts the main structural components of the blood brain barrier.

Mercury, another common toxic metal, crosses the blood brain barrier and can disrupt the function of the neurons, causing them to tangle together in clumps. When they are damaged in this way, the neurons cannot function properly. Alzheimer's patients have mercury blood levels at least three times higher than controls.

## Neurogenesis—Building New Brain Cells

Until the mid-sixties scientists generally believed we were born with a certain number of brain cells and that was it. If brain cells died or were damaged, there was no regeneration. Recent research indicates this is not true. The discovery was the result of happenstance. Elizabeth Gould, a professor at Princeton University's Department of Psychology, began investigating the effect of stress hormones on adult rat brains in 1989. To her surprise, while counting the dying brain cells, she observed new cells being created. This appeared to be a revolutionary idea, but it was not entirely new. In 1962 Joseph Altman, a scientist at MIT, had also found that rats, cats, and guinea pigs had formed new neurons. However, his findings were disregarded, and it wasn't until the late '80s, when other scientists found that neurogenesis occurred in fish, reptiles, and birds, that the idea took hold and scientists began to explore the human brain. Based on the work of Gould and others, a new field, neurogenesis, was created.

In support of this new field, scientists at the Karolinska Institute in Stockholm, Sweden, confirmed that adult humans showed substantial neurogenesis. Using retrospective carbon dating of human hippocampal cells from 55 deceased patients, who died between the ages of 19 and 92, Erickson and colleagues calculated that one-third of the neurons in the hippocampus, the area of the brain involved in forming, organizing, and storing memories, are regularly renewed throughout life. They calculated that roughly 1,400 new neurons were added per day, with rates declining modestly with age.

Other studies indicated that experiences and learning strengthened these new neurons, causing them to develop more dendrites and create more synapses. As the neurons were utilized, they developed more synaptic connections and became stronger. Those synaptic connections that were seldom used become weaker and died.

The foundation principles of neurogenesis are being used to develop new strategies for creating treatments from neurodegenerative diseases, such as Parkinson's, ALS, Alzheimer's, and multiple sclerosis. If the areas affected by these diseases could be made to produce new neurons, the symptoms of the diseases may be lessened or ameliorated.

The brain is also plastic. It can change its structure, a process known as structural plasticity, to accommodate experiences, exercise, dietary factors, drugs, disease, and brain injury. To maintain plasticity, neurons must be challenged and utilized through physical and mental exercise. As neurons are stimulated, the branches or dendrites grow outward into surrounding neurons, leading to better communication and better brain function. As communication improves between neurons, the brain becomes more efficient and functional. Even as we age and begin to lose some of the neurons over time, brain plasticity can still improve through ongoing stimulation. Healthy neuron connections support living to old age.

# Feeding and Care of Your Brain

As we age, there is a natural decline in overall brain function. Serious cognitive impairment, however, need not be considered part of normal aging. Numerous studies have shown that the symptoms of aging can be controlled. Staffan Lindeberg, in his book *Food and Western Disease: Health and Nutrition from an Evolutionary Perspective,* observed that adult-onset dementia was not found among the native populations of the Trobriand Islands and in East Africa. He concludes that dementia may not be a natural aging process. He also noted no strokes were reported among the native population in Papua New Guinea before 1975, and none were reported in Kenya or Uganda before 1940. As the countries became westernized, the incidence of stroke increased exponentially.

Another scientist, Dr. Gene Bowman at Oregon Health Sciences University, found study participants, with an average age of 87, with diets high in vitamins B, C, and E and omega-3 fatty acids were less likely to have brain shrinkage and other abnormalities associated with an increased risk for Alzheimer's disease. People whose diets were rich in those nutrients also had higher scores on cognitive functioning than people whose diets had fewer nutrients. They could think more clearly than those who consumed fewer nutrients. Dr. Bowman also found trans fats in baked goods and many processed foods, even in small amounts, were detrimental to cognitive functioning and brain volume.

Your brain needs basic nutrients from natural foods: carbohydrates, proteins, fats, vitamins, minerals, and water. Carbohydrates give the brain a steady supply of glucose, a major food for the brain. Proteins composed of amino acids build neurotransmitters and neurons. Good fat is needed to build cell membranes. Vitamins and minerals are essential nutrients that turn glucose into energy, amino acids into transmitters, and simple essential fats into more complex fats. Water makes up fifty-five to sixty percent of our total body mass and is necessary for all metabolic functions. To have a healthy brain, ingesting nutritious food, drinking water, and limiting toxins is necessary. The brain is an amazing organ. It requires and deserves the best of care.

# CHAPTER 5

# The Gut: Key to Health and Happiness

"THE ROAD TO GOOD HEALTH AND HAPPINESS IS PAVED WITH good intestines," Dr. T. R. LePine proclaimed in a presentation on the brain-gut connection. Although we are a nation obsessed with food—and eating—we seldom discuss how food is digested. Talking about our intestines or the elimination process is almost taboo in our culture. Our "gut" gets no respect, yet our physical and mental health depends on how well it functions. Eating nutritious food to maintain a healthy brain is important, but if the food isn't properly digested, the brain will not get the nourishment it needs, and your physical health, as well as your mental health, will suffer. "All diseases begin in the gut," according to Natasha Campbell-McBride, the creator of the GAPs Diet.

Although the gut is not honored, it truly is the key to good health and optimal brain functioning. Scientists are just beginning to understand just how elegant and complicated it is. Recent studies mapping all the microbes in the body have shown that of the 100 trillion cells in the body, only one in ten are actually you. The remaining cells are bacteria, viruses, and other microorganisms. Together, they are known as the microbiome. The microbiome resides on the surface and in deep layers of skin, in the saliva and oral mucosa, in the conjunctiva, and in the gastrointestinal tracts. Three and a half to four pounds of these microorganisms are found in the gut. There is 100 times more DNA in those microscopic organisms than in the cells of your body. But they're interdependent. The DNA in your body and the DNA in the microscopic organisms communicate with each other.

The digestive system, through a complicated and elegant process mostly orchestrated by these microbes, turns the food we eat into the microscopic nutrients that can be absorbed by the blood and carried to the cells throughout our bodies. The gut is the core of the immune system. It runs the metabolism, makes vitamins and hormones, produces clotting factors, metabolizes drugs, and helps remove toxins from the blood. The gut manufactures more neurotransmitters, like serotonin, than the brain. And it communicates with all the other cells in the body.

Unfortunately, our modern diet causes digestive problems, whether we talk about them or not. Findings from the Digestive Disease Clearinghouse and Information Center indicate that 60 to 70 million people are affected by all the digestive diseases, accounting for 104.7 million doctor visits in 2004 and costing the United States $141.8 billion in both direct and indirect costs.

Digestive problems are often the result of a poor diet. Bacteria, viral infections, injury, or disease can also cause digestive problems. A poor functioning liver or pancreas, two glands that promote good digestion, may exacerbate digestive problems as well. Recent research indicates the overuse of antibiotics may alter the gut microbiome and promote diseases. Chronic poor digestion can lead to malnourishment and the loss of amino acids, fats, and other nutrients. Thinking and memory can be impaired. If food is not properly digested and absorbed, diseases such as arthritis, autoimmune illness, fibromyalgia, chronic fatigue, or others may develop.

Eighty-five percent of the immune system is in the lining of the gut. The digestive system is made up of beneficial microbes and pathogens. As long as the beneficial microbes predominate, they control the pathogenic bacteria and viruses that live there. If the pathogens are out of control, they disrupt digestion and absorption. Rampant pathogens also damage the gut lining, creating a leaky gut. A leaky gut allows bad bacteria, viruses, and undigested food particles to circulate throughout the body, creating inflammation. Chronic inflammation may result if the immune system is continuously activated. Chronic inflammation in combination with a weakened body from poor digestion and absorption creates the conditions for all the major diseases, including brain disorders.

## How Digestion Works

Without healthy digestion and absorption we would languish and die. The digestive process actually begins with the brain. When we think about food, prepare it, smell it, and anticipate its flavor, our brains are getting our bodies ready. Our saliva begins to flow before we put anything into our mouths. As we start to chew, various enzymes and hormones from our salivary glands begin to digest the starches in our food. Thorough chewing allows food to be broken down into small particles so digestive juices in our mouths can do their work.

As food is swallowed, it moves through the throat into the esophagus, which connects the throat to the stomach. There are sphincters, ring-shaped muscles, at each end of the esophagus acting as gatekeepers, opening and closing to keep the food from flowing back into the esophagus or the throat. After the food passes through this tube, it enters the stomach, a bean-shaped, muscular organ, where food is stored and partially digested.

Hydrochloric acid, mucus, and enzymes secreted by the stomach lining are added to the food. Mucus, which coats the stomach lining, prevents the stomach from being damaged by the acids and enzymes. As the stomach's work is completed, the food, now a soupy goop, is slowly moved, through peristalsis, the involuntary contraction and relaxation of the digestive system, forward through the intestines.

Enzymes from the walls of the intestine continue the digestive process, preparing the food for absorption.

Carbohydrates, proteins, and fats are digested and broken down into their basic elements: carbohydrates into sugar, proteins into amino acids, and fats into fatty acids and glycerol. Carbohydrates are the most quickly digested because they are easily turned into glucose and absorbed. Proteins take a little longer, as acids and enzymes are required to dissolve the protein. Fats are the last to leave the stomach, because they are not water-soluble and require additional digestive enzymes to be converted into smaller particles.

The tiny capillaries in the intestinal wall absorb the nutrients as the food is digested. From the capillaries the nutrients move to bigger veins that join larger veins and eventually enter the liver through the portal vein. The portal vein drains the nutrient rich blood into the liver. The liver is the largest and perhaps most complex and hardworking organ in the body. Its main role is filtering the blood coming from the digestive tract before passing it to the rest of the body. The liver breaks down the nutrients in the blood so the body can use them and removes worn out cells, bacteria, and other foreign particles.

Bile, a fluid made by the liver and stored in the gallbladder, is vital to the digestive process. It contains mostly cholesterol, bile acids, and bilirubin (a breakdown product of red blood cells). During digestion bile is squeezed out through the bile ducts and into the intestines, where it assists in the digestion and absorption of fats. Bile is also responsible for the elimination of certain waste products from the body, like excessive cholesterol and destroyed red blood cells.

After being processed by the liver, most digested molecules of food are absorbed through the small intestine walls and moved in the blood throughout the body. The remaining waste products, largely undigested fiber, are moved into the large intestine or colon. Here, the final digestive processes take place. Bacteria in the colon synthesize vitamins B and K and metabolize bile. Some of the undigested fiber is converted into nutrients that nourish the colon cells.

The remaining material is stored as feces until a bowel movement pushes it from of the body. The journey from food to waste is a complex and miraculous process. However, digestion is more than movement of food through the digestive system. There is another layer of processing that gives us the energy for life.

## How the Body Turns Nutrients into Energy

When glucose molecules move from the bloodstream into the cells, the glucose needs to be converted into energy. Within each cell are thousands of smaller molecules called mitochondria. The mitochondria are the cells' energy factories. Mitochondria are semi-autonomous, because they are only partially dependent on the cell to replicate and grow. They have their own DNA and can make their own proteins. They turn the glucose from the digestive process into a substance called adenosine triphosphate (ATP). ATP is a high-energy compound that powers every one of our cells. The work that goes on within each of the 100 trillion human cells is because of the activity of 1 billion ATP molecules in each cell.

To create ATP, glucose needs oxygen. Respiration, or breathing, combines oxygen with glucose to create ATP. An end product, after the energy has been produced and expended, is the carbon dioxide that is breathed out. The ATP is second only to DNA in importance in how our bodies and brains function. The origin of ATP is the food we eat. Exercise, which increases the intake of oxygen through respiration, increases the production of ATP.

## The Gut, the Microbiome, and the Immune System

The intestinal walls contain two hundred times the surface area of the skin and are one of the first lines of defense against foreign invaders. The microbiome, made up of microorganisms, is located within the folds of the intestines. It makes up 85% of our immune system. If the intestines are healthy, populated with "good" microorganisms, they keep out foreign organisms and molecules. The cells on the walls of the intestine, through a scanning process of all cells they come in contact with, are able to determine if a cell is a friend or foe. If there is an invader, an undigested food particle, a toxin, or an unfriendly bacteria, the immune system is activated and goes to work. The components of the microbiome, the soldiers of the intestines, create inflammation to encapsulate, detoxify, or expel the invader.

The microorganisms that form the microbiome in the gut are passed down from generation to generation through vaginal birth. Nursing newborns promotes the growth of healthy microbiomes in their guts, but nursing may also account for how specific diseases are passed down through families. It is believed that changes in the microbiome change the expression of the genes and determine which genes are activated and which remain dormant.

The microbiome is just beginning to be understood. It was first identified in the late nineties. Since then, the microbiome has become the object of intense research and has led scientists to conclude that it may play a major role in health and in the development of diseases. Type 1 diabetes, an autoimmune disease, is correlated with an unstable gut biome. Gut microbes are also implicated in anxiety disorders, autism, and depression. Since some of the microbes in our bodies can modify the transmitters found in the brain, the microbiota may also have an effect on schizophrenia, bipolar disorder, depression, and other neurochemical imbalances.

Antibiotics can alter the gut microbiome. The Center for Disease Control reports that of the top ten prescribed drugs, five were antibiotics. In 2010, 8 out of 10 people were treated with antibiotics. Children by the age of two had received three courses of antibiotics. The destruction of parts of the microbiome by antibiotics appears to correlate significantly with the rise of obesity and may be implicated in other health-related issues. As the use of antibiotics has increased, there has been a corresponding rise in obesity. There is a surprising correlation, by state, of the rise of obesity and the increasing use of antibiotics.

Examining gut bacteria may lead to the identification of certain diseases. Scientists have found that people with a poor bacterial environment are more susceptible to type 2 diabetes. Research groups in Sweden compared the metagenome (a combination of human genes and the genes of the gut bacteria) of 145 women with type 2 diabetes with women who were healthy. By identifying the presence of altered gut microbes, they were able to predict which women were at risk for diabetes and which were not.

In an attempt to restore gut health for people with serious gut-related illnesses, a process called fecal microbiota transplant has been developed. It removes fecal matter from a person with a healthy gut and transplants it into the intestines of an ill person. Fecal microbiota transplantation is a way of recolonizing the gut flora with health-promoting microorganisms. And this may just be the beginning. As new research continues, scientists suspect that the gut microbiome may be responsible for many of the current maladies of our time. Understanding the gut microbiome's specific functions and manipulating them may reveal cures for many diseases.

## The Brain-Gut Connection

There is both an intimate connection between the brain and the gut and an almost completely separate connection. The brain-gut axis and the vagus nerve are the intimate connection; the gut as a second brain is the independent connection.

**The Brain-Gut Axis.** The brain-gut axis is the term used to describe the feedback loop between the digestive system and the brain. The two systems constantly exchange streams of chemical and electrical messages, working together to prompt the digestive process. The brain releases chemicals that tell the stomach when to produce acid, when to churn, and when to rest. The same signals tell the intestines when to release digestive enzymes and hormones.

In a feedback loop through the vagus nerve, the digestive system sends similar messages to the brain, creating sensations of hunger, fullness, pain, nausea, discomfort, and possibly, sadness and pleasure. The vagus nerve is a large cable that runs the length of the body. It originates in the brain stem and branches off into all the organs of the body. During the process of digestion, the brain activates the vagus nerve, which in turn, stimulates the intestinal muscles to digest and move food along the digestive tract.

Recent research has expanded the concept to the brain-gut axis to include the microbiome, so it has become the microbiome-gut-brain axis. As scientists learn more about the bacteria in the digestive tract, they are beginning to understand that bacteria are a third element in the communication system between the brain and the gut.

**The second brain.** One of the remarkable features of the gut is its ability to function independently of the brain. Unlike any other system in the body, it functions on its own as an intrinsic nervous system. The gut is able to mediate reflexes and control the movement and absorption of food through the intestines without input from the brain. If the connections between other parts of the body and the central nervous system are severed, as in a spinal cord injury, all reflex activity is terminated. However, even when serious brain injuries occur, people still get hungry, eat, digest, and eliminate food. All these functions continue because the gut has a mind of its own.

Our gut may also be the seat of our emotions. We know our digestive system is highly attuned to our feelings and states of mind. Butterflies in your stomach, a gut feeling, or the saying "go with your gut" are everyday examples of how we intuitively connect our feelings with our digestion. Science is affirming this folklore. Some researchers suggest that Prozac and other depressants actually work on the gut rather than on the brain. It is known, for example, that ninety-five percent of the serotonin, the feel-good neurotransmitter generally associated with the brain, is actually produced in the digestive system. Taken together, all the nerve fibers in the gut would be a mass larger than the mass of neurons in the brain. It is estimated that ninety-five percent of the nerve fibers in the vagus nerve go *from* the gut *to* the brain. The stimulation of the nerve fibers along this long pathway is believed to be responsible for most of our feelings.

When we are tired or stressed, we often reach for comfort food, such as macaroni and cheese, mashed potatoes, or ice cream. Our feelings create a craving for food that "comforts" us. An interesting experiment gives an underlying scientific reason why this might be so. Human volunteers were fed either a saline solution or an infusion of fatty acid via a nose tube so they couldn't identify what they were being fed. Then they were shown images of either sad or neutral faces and listened to either sad or neutral music. Based on both the reports of the volunteers' feelings and on brain images the researchers observed, the fatty acids reduced both sad feelings and sensations of hunger by half compared with the saline solution. The fat solution was comforting and satisfying. The scientists concluded that what we put in our guts might influence our moods, even in the absence of any pleasant associations we might have with the comfort food or the memories associated with it.

Other studies on mice came to similar conclusions, but with a slightly different twist. The mice were "bullied" by other creatures and then given a choice of peanut butter or their regular food. They preferred the peanut butter, a fatty, high-energy food. Scientists have begun to realize our emotions and our digestive systems are so closely related they are to be treated together for the most effective results.

# Causes of Poor Digestion

There are many ways digestion can be impaired or its function compromised. Some of the major culprits are leaky gut, chronic stress, candida, environmental contaminants, alcohol consumption, genetic modified organisms (GMOs), and poor food choices.

**Leaky Gut.** The small intestine has two functions, digestion and protection. If all goes according to plan, it allows digested nutrients from carbohydrates, proteins, and fats to pass from the intestine into the bloodstream. If there is an area of bowel inflammation, white blood cells encapsulate the affected area to form a barrier to prevent small nutrients and food molecules from passing through the wall of the intestine.

If the cells in the intestine become too damaged and the white blood cells can no longer create a barrier, then the gut leaks, a condition called leaky gut. Leaky gut is a breakdown of the tight junctures between cells in the lining of the gut. Bacteria and large food particles may pass from the intestine into the bloodstream, causing the body to develop antibodies to whatever substances have passed through. In addition to putting undue stress on the immune system, the antibodies cause food sensitivities, allergies, and increased sensitivities to environmental contaminants. Leaky gut has been implicated as an underlying cause of celiac disease, gluten sensitivity, Crohn's disease, HIV, asthma, bronchitis, psoriasis, rheumatoid arthritis, and other disorders.

A leaky gut may develop because of chronic stress, Candida, environmental contaminants, alcohol consumption, or poor food choices. The standard American diet, high in fast foods, processed foods, gluten, trans fats, and dairy, promotes a leaky gut. In other words, an inflammatory diet produces a leaky gut.

**Chronic stress.** Chronic stress takes its toll on our digestive systems by changing the composition, diversity, and number of gut bacteria. As the number of bacteria decreases, potentially harmful bacteria take over, affecting our immune systems and moods. Studies in mice suggest that chronic stress may also influence our personalities and our capacity for learning and memory. Scientists are exploring strategies for developing unique bacteria-based treatments for stress-related psychiatric disorders, such as anxiety and depression.

**Candida.** Candida is a systemic fungus that grows in the digestive system. It can weaken the immune system with an overgrowth of yeast. Candida feeds on simple carbohydrates and sugar in the gut.

It is believed to be the origin of many health problems, including fatigue, headache, poor memory, and weight gain.

**Environmental contaminants.** Toxins, household and industrial chemicals, air pollution, mold and fungus in our homes, and electropollution from cell phones and computer screens can all enter the body through the air we breathe and the items we touch. Each contaminant contributes to the disruption and suppression of the immune system.

**Alcohol consumption.** Consuming excessive alcohol is believed to suppress hormones in the gut, causing damage in the intestinal tract. It may also block the movement of nutrients from passing from the intestinal tract into the bloodstream.

**Consumption of GMO foods.** Genetically modified organisms have had an impact on our food supply. Most of the soybeans and much of the corn we consume comes from genetically modified crops. Most processed food, including beverages, contains GMOs. There is much debate about the effect of GMOs on our health, but digestive problems have increased as the amount of GM crops has increased.

**Poor food choices.** Poor food choices, such as low-fiber diets, highly processed food, food additives, trans fats, and sugar, promote inflammation in the gut. Low-fiber diets increase the transit time in the gut, allowing toxic byproducts to concentrate and irritate the gut lining. Highly processed foods contain chemicals and additives that are not natural food and that irritate the gut lining. Milk, grains, beans, and the disruption of the balance of the bacteria in the gut due to plant lectins can trigger autoimmune disorders caused by antigens.

**Other factors that damage the gut flora.** A modern day dilemma is our use of antibiotics, anti-inflammatory medications, aspirin, and other NSAIDs. They kill the bacteria that cause our illnesses, but they also destroy part of our microbiome. Our obsession with germs, cleanliness, and disinfectants, and the overuse of antibiotics can cause the whole microbiome in our guts to collapse. Without the ability to digest our food, we will perish.

# Love Your Gut

The digestive system is a highly complex mechanism, home to billions of bacteria, a second brain, and most of our immune system. When it functions well and the enzymes and microbes are in balance, our brains and bodies get the nutrients they need, and we are able to produce adequate ATP and function at maximum capacity. When digestive problems persist, our moods and our health are affected in a myriad of ways, from serious diseases to depression. As we learn more, the gut may become the new frontier for identifying and treating some diseases. Given all those complexities, much of our health and happiness really does depend on our guts.

# CHAPTER 6

# Chronic Inflammation: The Root of Disease

W E LIVE IN A WORLD THAT CHALLENGES OUR ABILITY AND motivation to maintain a healthy brain. Our food supply has been compromised by our need for a quick, easy meal and the producers' desire of profit. Food advertisements seduce us with beautiful images of delectable feasts. We love convenience foods full of tasty sugars, fats, and carbohydrates. Toxins are everywhere, in our food, in our homes, and in our neighborhoods. Our health is compromised by what we eat and where we live. As a result, our brains can suffer from chronic inflammation.

## Chronic Inflammation

Some inflammation is a good thing. When we break a bone, get a cut, burn ourselves, or are attacked by bacteria or viruses, the body's immune system kicks in. White blood cells, like good soldiers, flow through the affected area with their weapons of inflammatory compounds, destroying or killing the offending cells, picking up injured cells bodies, and repairing any damage that results. It's a microscopic battlefield. When the threat has been neutralized, anti-inflammatory compounds, like peace troops, turn off pro-inflammatory compounds, and the body's immune system returns to stasis. All is well on the cellular battlefield. This is an example of short-term inflammation.

However, short-term inflammation can turn into chronic inflammation. Chronic inflammation occurs when the pro-inflammatory response, the gung-ho soldiers, are not turned off. If the white blood cells from our immune response keep producing compounds to kill perceived invaders, the inflammation can become chronic. Injuries or chronic infections, certain foods, periodontal diseases, environmental toxins, and excessive free radicals cause chronic inflammation.

Severe chronic inflammation, as the origin of diseases, has just begun to be understood. When excess immune cells continue to flow through our systems, they damage blood vessel linings, brain neurons, joint tissue, gut mucosa, and pancreatic tissue, among many other body structures. It is now believed chronic inflammation is the root of most disease, contributing to dementia, Alzheimer's, atherosclerosis, diabetes, arthritis, celiac disease, Parkinson's, cancer, osteoporosis, autoimmune diseases such as rheumatoid arthritis and psoriasis, and other immune disorders.

## Causes of Inflammation

Causes of inflammation are everywhere. Some natural food products promote inflammation. Others create inflammation because of the additives they contain. Persons who are obese produce inflammation in their bodies from excessive abdominal fat. Periodontal disease creates inflammation that enters the bloodstream through our mouths. Pollution and toxins are ever present in our homes and neighborhoods. The more we understand the consequences of inflammation, the more critical it is to identify and remove the causes.

**Food related inflammation.** Dr. David Perlmutter, author of *Grain Brain*, is very clear about the role of food in overall health. He says, "You choose your level of inflammation very specifically by the foods you choose to consume." Although the USDA recommends making grain a part of our everyday diet, grain, particularly wheat, rye, and barley, contain the protein gluten. Gluten may trigger celiac disease, an inflammatory response in the lining of the small intestine, and gluten sensitivity, an inflammatory response that affects brain function. Lectin, another protein found in plants, is implicated in inflammation as well. Lectins are an important part of the plant's natural immune system and provide a protective barrier for the plant from invaders such as plant eaters, mold, or parasites. The body is unable to digest or destroy the lectin proteins because they are resistant to breakdown in the stomach or intestines.

Refined carbohydrates such as white bread, white rice, white potatoes, and foods that are primarily flour-based also contribute to inflammation by creating food sensitivities. Processed grains used in refined carbohydrates lose their fiber and much of their vitamin B and can hasten the onset of degenerative diseases. Food sensitivities can cause chronic inflammation, contributing to the deterioration of brain cells and the creation of brain lesions.

Feeding genetically modified corn and soybeans to commercially raised beef, pork, chicken, and farmed fish promotes inflammation in livestock. Adding antibiotics to fight infections from crowded conditions and growth hormones to promote accelerated growth further compromises our food. Traces of antibiotics and hormones remain in food products and are passed on to us. Processed meat such as sausages, salami, hams, and bacon may be even more problematic, and links have been found between processed meat and various cancers and heart disease.

Dairy products such as milk and cheese are allergens for as much as 60% of the world's population. Dairy can trigger inflammatory responses resulting in constipation, diarrhea, stomach distress, skin rashes, hives, and breathing difficulties.

Some fats, such as the polyunsaturated vegetable oils, safflower, corn, soybean, and peanut oils, contain high levels of omega-6 fatty acids. If a corresponding level of omega-3s is not present to balance omega-6s, chronic inflammation can occur. Trans fats, or partially hydrogenated oils, used in commercial baked goods and deep-fried foods also promote inflammation because of their unusual molecular structure. They increase bad cholesterol and cause obesity and insulin resistance. Trans fats also fundamentally change how the body metabolizes and stores fat.

Sugar has attained notoriety and is implicated in many major diseases. Historically, it has been held responsible for tooth decay, obesity, and type 2 diabetes. However, recent studies show that refined sugar may be a cause of cancer, lowered immune function, arthritis, cardiovascular disease, as well as diabetes. A diet high in sugar-sweetened soft drinks and foods rich in high-fructose corn syrup increases the biomarkers for inflammation in the blood.

Food additives may also cause inflammation as they break down into their chemical components and become toxic. Artificial sweeteners, MSG, food dyes, sodium nitrate and nitrite, and hundreds of other additives incorporated into food to preserve, enhance flavor, prevent spoilage, and act as filler also create an inflammatory response in our bodies.

**Obesity and chronic inflammation.** Unlike preventable diseases, such as diabetes and heart disease, that are the *result* of inflammation, obesity is a *cause* of inflammation. A high caloric diet provokes abdominal fat cells to act as if they are under attack, producing fat tissue inflammation that contributes to a range of diseases, including dementia and Alzheimer's.

Researchers at Johns Hopkins Bloomberg School of Public Health analyzed studies that included 37,000 people from the US, France, Finland, Sweden, and Japan. The findings showed that obesity increased the relative risk of dementia by an average of 42% when compared with normal weight. Specifically, obesity increased the risk of Alzheimer's up to 80% and the risk for vascular dementia by 73%. Being underweight increased the risk by 36%. The authors concluded that reducing the prevalence of obesity is a promising strategy for preventing the progression of normal aging into Alzheimer's disease.

**Chronic dental inflammation.** Periodontal disease is often overlooked as a source of chronic inflammation. The American Dental Association reports that 40% of the adult population has some form of periodontal disease. The percentage increases to 70% in adults over 65 years of age.

Periodontal disease is an infection of the gums and bones that surround and support the teeth. It's caused by bacteria and plaque buildup. Plaque, a sticky deposit around the teeth, can harden into tartar. As the tartar builds up, it causes the teeth to pull away from the gums, creating a pocket where more bacteria can grow. Chronic inflammation occurs when periodontal pockets become a home for anaerobic bacteria (bacteria the lives without oxygen). It is through these pockets that bacteria and their toxins enter the bloodstream, triggering an immune response that circulates throughout the whole body.

Gingivitis, an early stage of periodontal disease, is characterized by red, swollen gums. A later stage, periodontitis, indicated by periodontal pockets, leads to the loosening and loss of teeth. Chronic periodontal disease has been implicated in heart disease, strokes, respiratory diseases, kidney failure, and diabetes. The type of bacterium, spirochetes, implicated in these diseases is also found in the brains of Alzheimer's patients. A chronic spirochetal infection can cause dementia, brain atrophy, and amyloid deposition.

Mercury fillings are another source of inflammation. Used for decades, mercury fillings were determined by the Food and Drug Administration to be safe. In a recent turn around, the FDA has posted the following on its website: "Dental amalgams contain mercury which may have neurotoxic effect on the nervous systems of developing children and fetuses." The FDA also acknowledges that the fillings may release mercury vapor when placed in or removed from the teeth or when chewing. Some research suggests that mercury fillings may be linked to Alzheimer's and other diseases and disorders. Many European countries have banned or restricted the use of mercury in fillings.

**Free radicals and oxidation.** Technically speaking, a free radical is a molecule with one missing electron. The missing electron makes the molecule reactive and unstable, and it aggressively seeks to steal an electron from another cell, which in turn becomes reactive. Free radicals are produced when air is oxidized as we breathe. Normal cellular function causes the formation of free radicals. Free radicals help the immune system fight off diseases. However, too many free radicals can cause problems, because they "grab" electrons from adjacent molecules. If this occurs thousands of times and free radicals get out of control, cells will be damaged faster than they can be repaired. Brain neurons are especially vulnerable to free radical attacks. Free radicals wear out the maintenance mechanisms of the brain, causing the brain to age or reducing its ability to fight disease. Free radicals are involved in the degeneration of neurons in epilepsy, schizophrenia, tardive dyskinesia, normal aging, Parkinson's disease, and Alzheimer's disease. Free radicals have been implicated in accelerated aging, tissue damage in strokes, and the spread of cancer.

## Environmental Pollution

Toxins have become so much a part of our lives that we scarcely notice. They enter our digestive systems from food and our skin from air pollution. They invade our homes as molds and fungus. They are ever present in the products we use and as electropollution in our electronic devices. Toxins in our bodies are dangerous because they circulate in the blood and are stored in the brain and other major organs, where they create the conditions for disease. Toxins come in many forms.

**Air pollution.** People living in metropolitan cities may be exposed to severe air pollution that is a complex mix of gases, particulate matter, and organic compounds. Chronic exposure to severe air pollution creates inflammation common to the pathology leading to the formation of the plaques and tangles of Alzheimer's. Similar findings were suggested for people who were exposed to occupational and indoor air pollution.

**Product toxins.** Toxins in the form of polyvinyl chlorate (PVC) occur in new cars as hazardous flame-retardants, plasticizers, lead, and heavy metals used in armrests, dashboards, seats, and steering wheels. Another toxin, perfluorochemical (PFC), is found in the lining of grease-resistant food containers, microwave popcorn bags, and the lining of pizza delivery boxes. PFCs have been linked to low birth weight in newborns, elevated cholesterol, liver inflammation, and abnormal thyroid levels. Polybrominated diphenyl ethers (PBDEs) are a kind of toxic chemical found in computers, television screens, and carpet padding. PBDEs were linked to brain and nerve damage and are found in people of all ages, with babies and toddlers having three times the amount of their mothers.

Bisphenol A (BPA) is a common chemical found in clear, hard plastic bottles, sealable plastic bags, linings of aluminum soda cans, linings of steel cans that contain canned foods, medical devices, cash register receipts, and many other products. It is sometimes hard to isolate to truly determine its effect on human health. K. Kolber, writing in *Yale Environment 360* explains that when BPA comes in contact with heat or an alkaline environment, it changes chemically and becomes an active hormone. It is believed to be a contributing factor in heart disease, breast and prostate cancers, early puberty in girls, low sperm count, attention deficit hyperactivity disorder, learning disabilities, and many other disorders. It causes genes to reprogram. Fat cells also function differently in the presence of BPA and can promote obesity with *no* increase in caloric intake. The FDA does not stringently regulate BPA. It has been banned in Japan and is under investigation in Canada and the UK.

A Harvard School of Public Health study found the average newborn has 287 chemicals in its umbilical cord, 217 of which are neurotoxic. Infants are exposed to pesticides, phthalates, bisphenol A, flame retardants, and heavy metals such as mercury, lead, and arsenic. In addition to the broad range of negative effects on their little bodies and brains, the toxins appear to be causing obesity. The researchers noted that rates of obesity in infants less than six months old have risen 73% since 1980.

Another chemical, the ubiquitous Roundup, has been implicated in gastrointestinal disorders, obesity, diabetes, heart disease, depression, autism, infertility, cancer, Alzheimer's disease, Parkinson's disease, birth defects, and more. An April 2013 study in the journal *Entropy* found that glyphosate, which is also the active ingredient in several other brands of herbicides, disrupts the body's ability to detoxify foreign substances, such as pesticides, industrial chemicals, pollutants, and drugs. It disrupts the ability of intestinal microbes to manufacture important amino acids that build and repair cellular tissues. After reviewing 286 studies, the authors of the study, Samsel and Seneff, conclude, "Glyphosate may be the most biologically disruptive chemical in our environment." They urge more research to corroborate their findings.

**Household chemicals.** Household chemicals found in cleaners, solvents, pesticides, food additives, garden and lawn products, furniture, nonstick pans, and many other home products all contain toxins that can damage health. Vehicle exhaust, chemical pesticides, herbicides, petrochemical paints, and solvents also cause damage. Tobacco smoke, both firsthand and secondhand, is a major contributor to many diseases. The increase in toxins in the environment has also been implicated in the dramatic increase in diabetes. The cause is believed to be the disruption by toxins of the endocrine system.

**Molds and fungus.** Molds and fungus generate neurotoxins that are harmful. They grow in homes when the relative humidity goes over 40%. Molds and fungus cause asthma, chronic sinusitis, cognitive dysfunction, vision problems, chronic fatigue, fibromyalgia, rheumatoid arthritis, and many other diseases.

**Electropollution.** Electropollution, or dirty electricity, is the high voltage variation in current of the electrical wiring inside buildings. It is also produced by computers, television sets, entertainment units, dimmer switches, energy efficient appliances, and energy efficient wiring. Electrical pollution can also come from cell phones, cordless phones, chargers, modems, microwaves, and many other home appliances that we use every day. By some estimates, we are exposed, daily, to as much as 100 million times more electro-magnetic radiation than our grandparents were. According to radi-ationrescue.org, electropollution may also cause changes in blood sugar, DNA damage, suppression of the immune system, disruption of normal functioning of the neurological, cardiovascular, and endocrine systems, impaired cognitive functioning, and leakage in the blood brain barrier.

## Anti-Inflammatory Drugs

Nonsteroidal anti-inflammatory drugs (NSAIDs) are the pharmaceutical answer to inflammation. Each year over 70 million prescriptions are filled, and consumers make another 30 billion over-the-counter NSAID purchases. NSAIDs can be very effective in providing short-term relief from pain and inflammation. However, long-term use or exceeding the recommended dosage, particularly in Tylenol, can result in in serious side effects, including death.

Aspirin, ibuprofen, and naproxen are other over-the-counter NSAIDs that override the inflammatory response. Common names for these drugs, other than generic aspirin, are Advil, Motrin, Aleve, and others. The most common side effect of these drugs is stomach upset. Regular consumption can erode the stomach lining, causing inflammation of the stomach wall and the formation of gastric ulcers. NSAIDs are now the leading cause of ulcers. When used for joint pain, the regular use of aspirin and ibuprofen actually accelerates the breakdown of cartilage in joints.

Researchers Page and Henry found that seniors who used NSAIDs regularly and had a history of heart disease might have accounted for almost one-fifth of all hospital admissions for heart failure. A similar finding was published in *The Journal of the American Medical Association*, formerly *Archives of Internal Medicine*. The authors found that the regular use of NSAIDs, except for aspirin, doubles the risk of being hospitalized for heart failure.

Corticosteroids, a cortisone-like drug, the most common of

which is prednisone, is often prescribed by physicians to relieve the symptoms of autoimmune diseases such as multiple sclerosis, lupus, rheumatoid arthritis, and others. These drugs shut down the inflammatory response over time and have serious, long-term side effects. Because they reduce the action of the immune system, corticosteroids increase the body's susceptibility to infections and slow the healing of any wounds. They also interfere with the metabolism of necessary nutrients, leading to osteoporosis and contribute to elevated blood sugar, high blood pressure, coronary artery disease, loss of muscle mass, male infertility, cataracts, and glaucoma.

## Inflammation Dangers Are Everywhere

Immune systems need a balance between the pro-inflammatory and anti-inflammatory actions. To achieve this balance, we need to reduce our intake of trans fats, refined carbohydrates, and sugars. We need to reexamine our daily food intake to determine if grains, legumes, seeds, and milk need to be reduced or replaced. Sources of toxins, such as lead, mercury, and BPA, in our environment need to identified and avoided. Eliminating toxic cleaning chemicals, artificial fertilizers, and other toxins in our homes can also help protect our immune systems. Controlling inflammation is a challenging task in our modern world, but information is power.

SECTION THREE

# Feed Your Brain

CHAPTER 7

# Redeeming Fat

F AT, PARTICULARLY SATURATED FAT, HAS HAD A BAD RAP FOR
decades. But no matter what the "experts" say, it's essential for
good health. In addition to being critical for our brains, which are
60% fat, fat is the main fuel for our muscles, including the heart.
Fat is necessary for healthy liver and gall bladder function and for
the absorption of fat-soluble vitamins. It is required for the digestion of proteins. Stored fat enhances the function of the immune
system and helps fight infection. Fat cells produce hormones and
other compounds that affect metabolism, weight, and overall health.
Fat gives food flavor and makes it satisfying and tasty. If we have
enough fat in our diets, it reduces our craving for less healthy foods.

## The Myth of Fat and Heart Disease

In spite of all these vital functions, fat has had a bad reputation, particularly as a contributing factor to heart disease. Although there is
little scientific proof that a connection exists between fat consumption and heart disease, the USDA suggests that fat intake be limited.
Both the USDA's 2011 *MyPlate* and 1992 *Food Guide Pyramid* recommend limiting solid fats such as butter, milk fat, cream, beef fat,
pork fat, chicken fat, and coconut and palm oils, the very fats that
have been shown to promote brain health. To further discourage

consumers from eating saturated fats, the supplemental information for *MyPlate* lists many of the same fats, along with sugar, as "empty calories."

The USDA is not alone in their recommendations. Physicians, diet gurus, drug companies, and leading government health agencies are on the same bandwagon. They all recommend limiting fat intake by avoiding eggs, cheese, whole milk, red meat, and other foods that contain significant amounts of saturated fat. However, there is an enormous amount of solid research that indicates this link is a myth. George V. Mann, MD, of Vanderbilt University School of Medicine and Department of Chemistry (retired) and former director of the Framingham Heart Study says:

> For fifty years the public has been told by officials of the American Heart Association and the National Heart Institute that this epidemic [heart disease] is caused by dietary saturated fatty acids and cholesterol. That advice is quite wrong. It is the greatest biomedical error of the Twentieth Century. (Leas, p. 15)

Other research supports this statement. A recent meta-analysis of almost three hundred, fifty thousand subjects in twenty-one studies assessed the correlation between the consumption of saturated fats and cardiovascular disease and found that saturated fat was not associated with an increased risk of heart disease or stroke.

Nurses' Health Study II conducted by the Harvard School of Public Health accumulated over 10 years of data on diet and health from almost 300,000 Americans. The results suggest that the total fat consumed has no relation to heart disease risk. In an earlier report (1969), a distinguished panel of experts from the fields of medicine, nutrition, epidemiology, and metabolism concluded that changing eating patterns had no effect on heart disease. Furthermore, they reported that eating less fat could have a harmful effect on the body.

*The New England Journal of Medicine* published "Primary

Prevention of Cardiovascular Disease with a Mediterranean Diet" in February 2013, authored by scientists from Spain. A Mediterranean diet consists of a high intake of olive oil, fruit, nuts, vegetables, cereals, and sweets, plus wine consumed in moderation with meals. Their conclusions support the idea that good fat, in this case diets supplemented with olive oil (approximately 1 liter per week) and mixed nuts (30 grams per week), provide protection against coronary heart disease. Seven thousand, four hundred men and women between the ages of 55 and 80 with no cardiovascular disease at enrollment, but who had at least three major risk factors, such as diabetes, obesity, elevated LDL cholesterol levels, or a family history of premature coronary heart disease, participated in the study. The study participants showed a relative risk reduction in the rates of coronary heart disease of approximately 30%. The risk of stroke was also significantly reduced.

A study published in 2014 by Tulane University using a randomized trial with 148 obese men and women without cardiovascular disease or diabetes examined the effects of a low carbohydrate diet and a low fat diet on body weight and cardiovascular risk factors. The low carbohydrate group got 41% of their calories from fat, of which 13% was saturated fat. The low fat group included more grains, cereals, and starches in their diets and got less than 30% of their calories from fat. After a year the low carbohydrate group lost an average of 7.7 pounds more than the low fat group and had significantly greater reductions in body fat. The low carbohydrate group also had reduced markers for inflammation and triglycerides.

Other studies from around the world indicate fat is a necessary component of a healthy diet. For example, an Australian study followed subjects for fifteen years and found that people who ate the most full-fat dairy products had a 69% lower risk of cardiovascular death than those who ate the least. The people who mostly avoided dairy foods or consumed low-fat dairy had three times the risk of dying of coronary heart disease or stroke compared to people who ate the most full-fat dairy. A Japanese study found that saturated fat intake was inversely associated with mortality from stroke. In other words, those who ate more saturated fat were less likely to die from stokes. In the Seven Countries Study, US men had more than 100-fold higher incidences of coronary heart disease than Cretan men, despite identical fat intake, i.e., 40% of dietary intake. The amount of fat eaten was not a factor in their heart disease.

Greenland Eskimos and desert nomads, two very different populations, consume widely varied amounts of fat. The diet of the Eskimos consists of 50% fat; the desert nomads, 10% fat. These two disparate groups have the lowest rates of heart disease in the world. Another study indicated that the incidences of heart disease in Switzerland decreased after World War II, but the consumption of animal fat increased by 20%.

Fat is a critical component of the trillions of cells that are the building blocks of your physical self. How much body fat do you need? A typical healthy woman's body is about 25% fat; a typical healthy man's body is about 15% fat. About 60% of the brain is fat and brain fat has many critical functions. One of its most important functions is to build the cell walls of the brain. The brain has trillions of cells, and each cell, through its membrane or cell wall, is in constant communication and interaction with other cells. Through this communication and interaction, nutrients are provided, sugar and hormone levels regulated, new cells created, and detoxification occurs. In addition to all these functions, the brain cells are also responsible for concentration, memory, and mood. The health of our brains is very dependent on the quantity and quality of fat that we consume.

## The Cholesterol/Heart Disease Myth

Just as fat has gotten a bad rap, so has cholesterol. For years it was believed that saturated fat, those fats found in butter, animal fat, and dairy products, elevated blood cholesterol levels. The elevated cholesterol levels then led to arteriosclerosis, which increased the risk of heart attacks. In spite of millions of dollars spent on research to verify this hypothesis, the connection has never been thoroughly proven. Nor has the reduction in saturated fat consumption proven to extend a healthy individual's lifespan.

The authors of the Framingham Study, Herber and others, after 40 years of studying 6,000 people, found that the more saturated fat one ate, the more cholesterol one ate, the more calories one ate, the lower one's serum cholesterol. The authors reported that the people who ate the most cholesterol, ate the most saturated fat, ate the most calories, weighed the least, and were the most physically active. The Framingham Study began in 1948 with 5,209 participants. It has been followed by the Offspring Study (with spouses) and the Third Generation Study.

Other research suggests the following: People with higher blood cholesterol have been found to be capable of faster mental processing than those with low cholesterol, and that those whose levels of blood cholesterol are unusually low, or have been artificially reduced, seem to be more prone to suicide and aggressive behavior. Additional studies indicate:

- Half the people who have heart attacks and strokes do not have high blood cholesterol.
- People whose blood cholesterol is low develop just as many plaques in their blood vessels as people whose cholesterol is high.
- Older women with high cholesterol live longer than older women with low cholesterol.
- Cholesterol levels do not predict the risk of a heart attack in men over age sixty-five.

In the 34-year follow-up of the Framingham studies, high cholesterol was not predictive of heart disease after the age of 47. In fact, the studies showed that those over 50 whose cholesterol went down had the highest risk of having a heart attack. However, high total cholesterol has been shown to be a risk factor for coronary heart disease in young and middle-aged men. One explanation is that men of this age are in the midst of advancing their professional careers and are therefore more acutely stressed than other age groups. Mental stress is a well-known cause of cardiovascular disease.

**LDL and HDL, the magic numbers.** Cholesterol is made up of fats and oils called lipids that cannot dissolve in the bloodstream. Carriers in the blood called lipoproteins transport the lipids throughout the body. Two of the lipoproteins are LDL, low-density lipoproteins (small, dense particles of cholesterol), and HDL, high-density lipoproteins (larger particles of cholesterol). Higher numbers of LDL are associated with increased risk of coronary heart disease. When there is inflammation or injury, because of their size, the LDL particles lodge themselves more easily than larger HDL particles into arterial walls, causing plaque buildup and cell wall damage. Oxidation of the LDL molecules in the blood vessel walls is thought to cause hardening of the arteries. HDL is associated with a decreased risk of coronary heart disease, because they are less likely to lodge themselves into arterial walls.

In a Swedish study that followed 175,000 patients with heart disease, researchers found that they were three times more likely to have larger numbers of LDL than HDL. Low-fat, high-carbohydrate diets have consistently been shown to create the smaller, denser, more dangerous particles (LDL). Low-carbohydrate, higher-fat—especially saturated fat—diets create larger cholesterol particles (HDL) and are less likely to contribute to heart disease. Although lowering LDL appears to be a factor in decreasing the risk of heart disease, recent research indicates that raising the HDL does not reduce the risk of heart disease.

The issue of cholesterol is very complex, and more information about HDL and LDL is appearing in the literature. Dr. Mark Houston, author of *What Your Doctor May Not Tell You about Heart Disease*, states, "Cholesterol is *not* inherently bad, and an elevated level is not a sure sign of coronary heart disease—anymore than low levels are a promise of heart health." (p. 62) He explains that HDL cholesterol comes in at least five different forms, and they change shape and size depending on the role they are called upon to play. Some forms are more protective than others. The kind and amount of HDL you have is more important and predictive than your overall number. The same is true of LDL cholesterol. There are three different forms of LDL. Each is more or less dense depending on their composition. It is the smallest that is the most dangerous, because it can slip through the walls of the endothelium and burrow into the arterial walls, beginning the inflammatory cascade that can lead to a stroke or heart attack.

**Benefits of saturated fat and cholesterol.** A 1992 analysis found that low intakes of saturated fat and dietary cholesterol were associated with small, dense LDL particles. Men eating less saturated fat and less total fat were more likely to have high rates of stroke. The total intake of fat, saturated fat, monounsaturated fat, and polyunsaturated fat was associated with reduced risk of ischemic stroke in both sexes.

The Framingham Study linked low cholesterol with greater risk of cancer. Women ages 56 to 70 had the lowest mortality rates when their total cholesterol was between 240 and 280 milligrams/deciliter (mg/dL). Women over 70 with cholesterol levels under 240 mg/dL had greater mortality rates.

Another study provides a cautionary note. The Northern Manhattan Study was composed of a diverse group of participants. The mean age was 69. It included 63% women, 21% white, 24% black, and 52% Hispanic. The results suggest that increased daily total fat intake for this diverse group, *above 65 grams,* significantly increases risk of ischemic stroke.

**Cholesterol serves vital functions.** Cholesterol is a steroid alcohol manufactured in the liver and in most cells. The major part of circulating serum cholesterol is produced by the liver, rather than absorbed from food. Cholesterol plays a vital role in keeping our cells healthy and does the following:

- Provides the precursors to make phospholipids, a fatty compound that makes up much of the brain

- Gives cell membranes their necessary structure
- Acts as an antioxidant protecting cells from free radicals
- Is the natural healing substance that repairs the damage when free radicals or viruses damage blood vessels or if there is an excess of polyunsaturated fats in cell membranes
- Functions as a component of bile, needed for the digestion of fat
- Is necessary for all hormone production
- Facilitates many biochemical processes, including mineral metabolism, blood sugar regulation, and the synthesis of hormones
- Is needed by the receptors in the brain to properly utilize the "feel good" chemical serotonin to maintain a healthy nervous system

# What Really Causes Heart Attacks and Strokes?

There is disagreement in the medical and scientific community about what causes cardiovascular disease. The commonly held notion that elevated cholesterol, high blood pressure, diabetes, obesity, and smoking are the primary causes of heart disease has been called into question by new research. While these factors play a role, new findings indicate that heart disease and strokes actually originate in the endothelium of the blood vessels. The endothelium is the smooth lining of the blood vessels, is one cell thick, and is the interface between the blood and the blood vessel.

The endothelium is considered a major organ and is the brain of the arteries. It functions to:

- Be a barrier and allow only certain substances to pass from the blood into the artery
- Regulate the immune system within the artery
- Regulate blood pressure
- Control inflammation and oxidation stress

- Maintain homeostasis within the blood
- Regulate the viscosity of the blood
- Control blood clotting

Heart disease occurs when the endothelium is disrupted by inflammation and one or more of these functions are disrupted. Endothelium inflammation is caused by a number of factors, including chronic infections, oxidation of LDL cholesterol, elevated levels of glucose, toxins, heavy metals, cigarette smoke, or excessive stress. As with all inflammations, the immune system responds and sends white blood cells, platelets, and other immune cells to repair the damage. If the damage repair is incomplete or ineffective, other cells and particles can seep through the endothelium and into the arterial wall. As more white blood cells and platelets are released to augment the repair process, the patch gets bigger. The "patch," or plaque buildup, on the artery wall from the inflammation response can continue to gather other immune cells and debris that stick to the artery wall. As it grows larger, it may erupt and discharge all the material into the bloodstream. This eruption can cause excessive clotting that may result in a heart attack or stroke.

This is a simple explanation for a very complex process called endothelium dysfunction. LDL is one contributor to the process of plaque buildup in the arteries. When there are high levels of LDL in the blood, it is believed that some may build up at the site of the inflammation. The inflammation attracts certain kinds of white blood cells that also stick to the walls of the arteries, causing other cells to grow around it, and if the process continues, plaque can form. It is this plaque, at the site of an inflammation, that is the source of concern. However, inflammation in the endothelium is the primary cause of the process, not the cholesterol buildup. The cholesterol buildup is a contributing factor.

A recent article in the British journal *The Lancet* added detailed scientific information to the process. The authors described a collaborative study among 43 research institutions around the world examining the cause of heart disease and probable drugs to target the disease. The lead author, Daniel Swerdlow, is quoted as saying:

> Previous studies have shown an association between inflammation and the risk of heart attacks, but until now there has been no direct evidence of a cause-effect relationship. Here we show that the IL6 receptor (IL6 is a protein complex that regulates cell growth and plays an important role in immune response) play a pivotal role in the development of coronary heart disease.

**Effects of cholesterol lowering drugs.** Statin drugs, such as Lipitor and Pravachol, are widely prescribed to combat high cholesterol. The drugs inhibit an enzyme that is required in the production of cholesterol. In doing so, they cause serious side effects by inhibiting the synthesis of other enzymes that build and regulate cells.

Although statin drugs are one of the most widely prescribed medications, they have proven to only slightly lower mortality in trials for men with the highest risk for heart disease. One trial (CARE, Cholesterol and Recurrent Events) with 4,000 people ages 21 to 75 with a past history of heart disease, indicated that for people who took a placebo, the odds of escaping death from a heart attack in five years was 94.3%. For those who took the statin drug, the odds improved to 95.4%.

There are many side effects to taking statin drugs, and careful consultation with a knowledgeable doctor is highly recommended before beginning the lifelong commitment. Some of the side effects include:

- Muscle weakness
- Liver and nerve damage
- Rhabdomyolysis: Muscle fibers break down and are released into the bloodstream, which may result in kidney failure
- Problems with memory, depression, and irritability
- Headaches
- Joint and abdominal pain

- Tingling and numbness of extremities
- Problems with sleeping
- Sexual dysfunction
- Fatigue, dizziness, and a sense of detachment

## Good Fat, Bad Fat

The USDA suggests we consume less than 10% of our calories from saturated fatty acids and less than 300 milligrams per day of cholesterol. They recommend total fat consumption make up between 20 and 35% of our diet. Although these are reasonable numbers (a minimum of 30% fat is required for good health), the recommendations are accompanied by the admonitions to choose meat, poultry, milk, and milk products that are lean, low-fat, or fat-free and to avoid eggs. Where will the good fat come from? Fat can come from olive oil and nuts, but to consume an adequate amount of fat, the fats must come from some of the same foods the USDA suggests we avoid. However, it is important to eat the right kind of fats.

The difference between good fats and bad fats is in their molecular makeup and how they are processed. Healthy fats are those used in their natural states, raised under natural conditions, or extracted from their source with minimal processing. Animal fat, like the fat in a beefsteak or a pork chop, is fat that does not need to be processed. Butter is an example of a fat that is minimally processed. It needs to be separated from raw milk. Olive oil is another example of fat that is minimally processed. It needs to be extracted from olives. The essential nature of these fats is not changed in the minimal processing.

On the other hand, bad fats, hydrogenated fats or trans fats, are vegetable oils that are highly processed to make them solid or to increase their shelf life. They are used in margarines, some vegetable cooking oils, for frying fast foods, and in commercial baked goods such as cake and cookies. Hydrogenated or trans fats are usually heated to a very high temperature and a hydrogen atom is added. The practice changes the molecular structure of the fat. The fats found in processed food, heated vegetable oil, processed vegetable oils, and hydrogenated fats can make the membranes of nerve cells rigid and unresponsive, leading to impaired nerve function, brain inflammation, and degeneration and other symptoms of impaired bran function.

Fats are generally grouped into four categories based on their molecular structure. The kinds of fat are:

- Saturated fats
- Monounsaturated fats
- Polyunsaturated fats
- Trans fats

All fats are combinations of one or more of the above. For example, olive oil, one of the healthiest fats, is composed of 13% saturated fat, 74% monounsaturated fat, and 8% polyunsaturated fat. Butter is 62% saturated fat, 29% polyunsaturated fat, and 8% polyunsaturated fat. A mixture of fats in your diet is necessary to maintain maximum health. The exception is trans fats, which should be avoided, unless they occur naturally in food products.

**Saturated fats.** Saturated fats are highly stable, solid or semi-solid at room temperature, and maintain their freshness with proper use. They do not become toxic at high temperatures.

Saturated fats, like other kinds of fat, are composed of many different fatty acids. All are necessary for your body to perform certain functions and to make use of vitamins and minerals. Saturated fats are easily broken down and used as energy. Fats not utilized are stored as fat tissue. Some of the saturated fats function as antibacterial and antiviral agents and have been shown to prevent tumors. They are the preferred nutrient for the brain and the heart. Saturated fat comes from either animal sources like poultry, beef, pork, and some fish, or in products like butter, milk and eggs. Plant sources include coconut and palm oil and avocados.

**Monounsaturated fats.** Monounsaturated fats are oils that become solid when refrigerated. Olive oil is the most common monounsaturated fat and is widely used for its taste and healthful properties. It's primarily oleic acid, which scientists have discovered has naturally occurring anti-inflammatory qualities.

Safflower and sunflower oils, if genetically modified, are also monounsaturated fats. Both contain high levels of omega-6 fatty acids, which when combined with omega-3 fatty acids in proper proportions, are essential to maintaining a healthy body and brain. These oils are not recommended for an anti-inflammatory diet.

Canola oil is also a common source of monounsaturated fat, but is also not recommended. Because canola oil becomes smelly and easily rancid when exposed to oxygen and high temperatures, it must be deodorized. The deodorization process removes much of the good fats and turns them into trans fats. Research studies indicate that canola oil may inhibit growth and cause fibrotic lesions in the heart and vitamin E deficiencies. The Food and Drug Administration does not allow canola oil to be used in infant formulas.

Significant amounts of monounsaturated fats occur in chicken, duck, goose, and turkey fat, lamb, bacon, lard, avocados, and almond butter.

**Polyunsaturated fats.** Polyunsaturated fats are primarily composed of two fatty acids: omega-3 fatty acids and omega-6 fatty acids, called essential fatty acids. Unlike most other fats, our bodies cannot synthesize these fatty acids and so must get them from the food we eat, therefore the name "essential." Omega-6s are most commonly found in sunflower oil, sesame oil, corn oil , peanut oil, safflower oil, soybean oil, and other vegetable oils. Omega-3s are found in fish and fish oil, flax seed oil, wheat germ, walnuts, and almonds.

Omega-3 and omega-6 fatty acids are vitally important, as they are part of the soft membranes around our cells that allow nutrients, vitamins, hormones, and messages to be transmitted between cells. They also serve complementary functions that work in tandem with each other. For example, omega-3s lower blood pressure and omega-6s raise blood pressure. Their synergy helps maintain balance in brain and body function.

Research suggests the consumption ratio of omega-6s to   should be 1:1 or 2:1. Because Americans have reduced their consumption of omegas-3s, found in butter, red meat, and eggs, and increased their consumption of omega-6s through eating processed foods and poly-unsaturated vegetable oils, the current ratio for consumption of ome-ga-6s to  in the United States ranges from 10:1 to 20:1, far out of line for a healthy body and brain. For this reason, it is important to limit consumption of polyunsaturated oils.

Omega-9s, another very important fatty acid, unlike  and ome-ga-6s, is available in foods and is one of the most abundant in nature, and therefore, is not considered an essential acid. Omega-9 fatty acids can be used by the body as a substitute for  and omega-6s if the others aren't present. However, this is not an ideal situation. Omega-9s are found in animal fats and vegetable oils and particu-larly in olive oil as oleic acid.

Although polyunsaturated fats are the source of  and omega-6s, they have another function that sets them apart from the healthful qualities described above. They are used to create trans fats.

**Trans fats.** Trans fats, often labeled as partially hydrogenated oil, are manufactured from polyunsaturated fats using pressure, high heat, and industrial solvents. During the process of changing the polyunsaturated fats to trans fats, the molecular structure is altered to make them highly stable. Trans fats may also be labeled vegetable shortening or shortening, and are made from soybean, canola, palm, cottonseed, corn, or safflower. Products like margarine or other butter substitutes are also made from polyunsaturated or trans fats. Most partially hydrogenated oils are made from soybeans, but regardless of the source, they are bad for your brain health.

Partially hydrogenated fats, or trans fats, are difficult for the body to use. Because their molecular form is changed during manu-facturing, they do not fit receptor molecules in the cell walls, thereby weakening the cell walls and allowing unwanted substances to enter the cell. They also cause the cell membranes to become hard and inflexible, inhibiting the communication between cells. Trans fats affect the immune system by reducing the capacity of the cell mem-branes to respond to injury or infection.

Trans fats also cause inflammation by promoting the production of chemicals that cause oxidation and structural damage to cells, including neurons and endothelium cells. Chronic inflammation in the brain can result in problems of cognition, depressive symptoms, and anxiety. Compared to saturated fats, trans fats increase the risk of diabetes and cardiovascular blockage by more than tenfold. Trans fats have a half-life of 51 days. This means that once you have eaten a product containing trans fat, the trans fat will stay in your body for 102 days, causing the problems to the brain that are described above. Trans fats must now be labeled on food packages. The FDA has finally proposed legislation that will limit the use of trans fats in food processing. It is not yet law.

Because of the negative publicity generated by trans fats, a new substitute has been developed by the food industries called interesterified fats. These fats not only raise LDL (the "bad" cholesterol) and lower HDL (the "good" cholesterol), as trans fats do, they also appear to raise blood sugar by 20 to 40%. Higher blood sugar is a precursor to diabetes. Because it is a new product, it has not been widely researched and has no rating by the FDA.

Not all trans fats are bad. Small amounts occur naturally in the meat and/or milk of cows, goats, and sheep. Lard, a solid or semi-solid fat obtained by rendering and clarifying the fatty tissue of a hog, is also a healthy source of trans fat. These trans fats are not processed like the hydrogenated oils and shortening and have been found to have anticarcinogenic properties. In a study conducted on the island of Okinawa, where the average lifespan for women is 84 years, the islanders eat large amounts of pork and fish and do all their cooking in lard. In other words, limited amounts of trans fats, if they occur in nature, may be good for you.

## Cooking with Fats and Oils

Each fat or oil has a different smoke point, or temperature at which it begins to smoke. A fat or oil heated to the smoking point breaks down and becomes toxic. Smoke points vary depending on how the fat or oil is processed. The smoking temperatures below are averages and approximations. For example, extra virgin oil has a smoke point of 406°F. Extra light olive oil has a smoking point of 468°F. Here are general guidelines for using fats and oils and their smoking points.

**Butter** is best used to enhance the flavor of baked goods and vegetables, and as a spread for bread. It needs to be refrigerated to preserve its flavor. Butter can be used for low heat sautéing and is more versatile for that purpose if combined with olive oil. Smoke point: 275°F

**Ghee**, which is butter that has been slowly heated until the milk solids separate, can be used for frying. Smoke point: 482°F

**Lard** has a relatively high smoke point and is especially useful for cooking and frying. Smoke point: 400°F

**Olive oil** can be used for salad dressings, on bread and vegetables, and for cooking at low to moderate temperatures. It is the most versatile of all vegetable oils. Smoke point: 325°F

**Coconut oil** has antifungal and antimicrobial properties, and if refined, can be used for cooking and frying. Smoke point: unrefined 280°F/refined 450°F

**Peanut oil (refined)** can be used for high temperature frying, but because it has a high percentage of omega-6s, it is not recommended for cooking. Smoke point: 450°F

**Non-hydrogenated palm oil** is stable at room temperature and has health supporting properties. It can be used for cooking and frying. Smoke point: 455°F

**Flaxseed oil** is valued for its high content of . It should always be refrigerated, never heated, and used only for salad dressings and spreads. Smoke point: 225°F

**Sesame oil** can be used for cooking and frying but contains high levels of omega-6s. It is not recommended for cooking. Smoke point: 450°F

*Note: Duck, goose, and chicken fat are also recommended for frying, although they are seldom available commercially. Many chefs at high-end restaurants report using duck or goose fat for preparing their gourmet foods.*

*Generally speaking, all cooking oils and fats are best used at the lowest possible temperature to preserve their nutrients and prevent oxidation.*

## Nuts: A Nutrient-Dense Food

Nuts (tree nuts and peanuts) are often overlooked as an excellent source of unsaturated fatty acids. Nuts have a total fat content ranging from pistachios at 76% to cashews at 46%, making them the natural plant food richest in fat after vegetable fats. Chestnuts, which have little fat, are an exception. Nuts contain a combination of unsaturated fat and monounsaturated fatty acids in combination with polyunsaturated fatty acids. They are one of our healthiest foods. Walnuts, particularly, as a whole food have the highest content of plant omega-3 fatty acids of all edible plants.

Many diet plans suggest limiting nut intake. However, extensive research shows that nut consumption is associated with reduced incidences of coronary heart disease and gallstones, and has positive effects on blood pressure, visceral adiposity, and the metabolic syndrome. Nuts have a beneficial effect on oxidative stress, inflammation, and vascular reactivity. Epidemiologic studies and clinical trials suggest that regular nut consumption is unlikely to contribute to obesity or diabetes and may even help in weight loss. Both the USDA and the American Heart Association have recommended that nuts be included as part of a healthy diet for health promotion and disease reduction. Ideally, nuts should be soaked before consumption to reduce the amount of phytic acid and other antinutrients found in their coatings.

## The Role of Omega-3 Fatty Acids in Brain Health

Omega-3 fatty acids are called essential fatty acids because they are not made by the body and must be consumed in our food. Two crucial essential fatty acids, eicosapentaenoic acid (EPA) and docosahexaenoic acid (DHA), are found primarily in certain fish. Alpha-linolenic acid (ALA), another omega-3 fatty acid, is found in plant sources such as nuts and seeds. EPA is necessary to promote cardiovascular health and optimum cell membrane development and maintenance. DHA is critical for the development of the brain, eyes, and autoimmune system. Omega-3s can also promote the genetic expression of a chemical known as brain-derived neurotrophic factor (BDNF), or nerve growth factor. This nerve growth factor contributes to the growth, integrity, and maintenance of the adult nervous system.

There is much evidence that omega-3 fatty acids can improve brain function and overall health, promoting a longer, healthier lifespan. A Nobel Prize was awarded to a team of Scandinavian scientists who studied the effects of omega-3s on Icelanders, to whom fish is a diet staple. The Icelanders were 20 times more likely to live longer than Americans—and do so in good health. The Icelanders have less heart disease, less high blood pressure, and fewer stokes than any other nationality in the world. They are also relatively free of depression. Icelandic women have a very low rate of infant mortality and give birth to infants having very advanced immune and nervous systems and exceptional brain and eye development.

As in the case of Islandic infants, there is considerable evidence linking intake of omega-3s with early brain development (prenatal to adolescence). Studies have also shown there is a positive relationship between higher levels of DHA in middle adulthood (between ages 35 and 55) and better cognitive functioning, including nonverbal reasoning, mental flexibility, working memory, and vocabulary. A similar finding was reported in a study in elderly men between the ages of 70 and 89. The authors concluded that a moderate intake of DHA/EPA from fish might postpone cognitive decline in elderly men.

The total brain is composed mostly of fat and requires five times more omega-3s than the red blood cells. If fatty acids are not available, other less effective fatty acids are used, most commonly, omega-6s.

When this substitution occurs, the cell walls, the transmission of signals, the uptake of serotonin and other neurotransmitters, the fluidity of the synaptic membranes, and almost all other brain functions are compromised. Omega-3 deficiency also leads to a breakdown in the normal functioning of the blood brain barrier, which allows chemicals that are normally excluded to enter the brain.

Our bodies and brains also need omega-3s to counterbalance the high levels of omega-6s in our modern diet. Omega-3s reduce the chronic inflammation that is a reliable predictor of brain dysfunction. They fight the inflammation that results from the pollutants and toxins in our environment. There is a growing body of evidence that shows without adequate amounts of omega-3s, some people may be at greater risk for depression, bipolar disorder, schizophrenia, and other psychiatric disorders. It is interesting to note that the increase in depression since 1954 coincides with the mass introduction of omega-6 fatty acids in the form of inexpensive vegetable oils.

According to Michael Schmidt, author of *Brain-Building Nutrition: How Dietary Fats and Oils Affect Mental, Physical, and Emotional Intelligence*, there are more than 50 conditions of the brain that involve fatty acids or have responded to fatty acids. His conclusions are based on the review of several thousand research papers, lab reports, and magnetic resonance imaging (MRI) reports. Some of the conditions that have responded positively to fatty acids are Alzheimer's disease, autism, bipolar disorder, chronic fatigue, memory problems, learning disabilities, schizophrenia, stroke, tremors, and violence.

DHA has implications for mental health status. Low DHA has been found among men in prisons who were described as violent and antisocial. High intake of linoleic oil, a component of omega-6s, has also been associated with higher levels of homicide rates in Argentina, Australia, Canada, the United Kingdom, and the United States. High intake of omega-6s was also implicated in higher rates of suicide, domestic violence, and depression.

**Omega-3s and mental functioning.** The Icelandic Longevity Institute has gathered studies showing that fish oil has large quantities of the essential fatty acids EPA and DHA. Countries with the highest rates of fish eating had the lowest rates of depression. Studies from Japan where people in villages eat high amounts of fish, incidences of depression were very low—ten times lower than in the United States. Here is a sample of other studies indicating the effect of omega-3s on mental health:

- Prescribing fish oils, flax oil, and omega-3 supplements has successfully treated bipolar disorder, depression, and other mental illnesses.
- Omega-3 fatty acids reduce anxiety in otherwise healthy adults.
- Fish oil has been effective in relieving childhood depression. Children who received fish oil capsules significantly improved their rating on the Childhood Depression Rating Scale.
- Omega-3 fatty acids possess powerful antiarrhythmic properties and may be effective in treating both major depression and sudden cardiac death, two conditions that have recently been associated with each other.
- There is considerable evidence that cell membrane structure is a significant factor in depression. This structure, in turn, is highly dependent on the presence of DHA. Scientists in the United Kingdom have found the severity of depression to be inversely proportional with the red blood cell level and dietary intake of omega-3 fatty acids.
- New studies have indicated schizophrenia is associated with an abnormal metabolism of unsaturated fatty acids in both blood plasma and red blood cells. This abnormality, in turn, is associated with very low levels of EPA, DHA, and arachidonic acid (AA) in cell membranes. The supplementation of omega-3 fatty acids, which increases the levels of DHA, EPA, and AA, has been shown to reduce the symptoms of the disease.
- Daily vitamin and a fish oil supplements (compared with two placebos) reduced violent acts for young offenders by 37% within a UK prison. When the trial was completed

and the supplements stopped, the offenses returned to the previous levels.

The importance of omega-3s in brain health is not completely accepted in the medical community. Because there is not a one to one correlation between mental functioning, psychiatric disorders, and omega-3 deficiencies, omega-3s are not prescribed as part of a comprehensive health/treatment plan. It is an over-the-counter product and not available through drug company representatives, who are often the source of information for traditional providers. Our modern diet does not provide enough omega-3s, but they can be added through the supplementation of fish oils.

## Are Fish Oils Safe?

There are some reports that unpurified fish oil may contain Mercury, PCBs, and/or dioxins. To address this issue, the Environmental Defense Fund (EDF) conducted a survey of major producers and suppliers of fish oil supplements in the United States to see if and how they were addressing the health risks from these and other contaminants. Of the 75 companies contacted, more than 80% (61) verified they had met the strictest US standards.

The Food and Drug Administration, the US Environmental Protection Agency (EPA), the Canadian Food Inspection Agency, the European Union, and the State of California (Proposition 65) set the standards considered in the survey. The EPA and California had the most stringent standards, so they were chosen to evaluate the fish oil products. The Environmental Defense Fund concluded their investigation with this statement: "In short, most fish oil supplements appear to be adequately purified and safe. Consumers who take fish oil should consider purchasing them from companies that verified they have met the strictest US standards for contaminants." Molecular distillation techniques allow fish oils to be gently purified so they are not damaged, yet heavy metals, such as mercury, PCBs, and other toxins, are removed to below detectable limits.

Fish oil supplements are made from small species of fish, such as anchovies, sardines, mackerel, and menhaden. Although these fish reproduce quickly and are caught by methods that do not imperil other marine life, they are important to the food chain, and standards for catch limits need to be considered. Omega-3 supplements can also be plant-based from flaxseed oil, but these are not as easily absorbed by the body. They also lack the fatty acids EPA and DHA. Marine algae, a good source of DHA, which can be raised in land-based tanks, may be the dietary supplement of the future. The American Heart Association in an AHA Scientific Statement recommends plant-based omega-3 over fish-based omega-3s, due to the toxins, particularly mercury, found in some fish.

Most commercial producers of omega-3 oils are certified for the purity of their ingredients and indicate where the fish come from. However, some oxidation may occur as the fish oils are processed. Vitamin E is often added to counteract this effect. Some studies recommend supplementing 200 milligrams of vitamin E with fish oil to assure the level of vitamin E in the body remains stable. Consult your medical provider before taking large doses of fish oil supplement.

**Other sources of omega-3s.** Omega-3s are also found in free-range beef, pork, lamb, poultry, dairy products, and specialized eggs. Vegetable sources provide ALA, which is converted to DHA or EPA. ALA is found in the oils of flaxseeds, canola, soybeans, walnuts, and some green vegetables, such as Brussels sprouts, kale, spinach, and salad greens. For vegetarians, algal derived DHA supplements are available.

## What Shall We Do?

Although it is very difficult to go against the recommendations of the USDA and the powerful medical establishment, there is a growing body of evidence that indicates it is our Western diet causing many of our health problems. It is not the saturated fats. It is the polyunsaturated fats, the trans fats, and the processed foods that are the guilty parties—along with our sedentary lifestyles. Good fats are important for our overall health and critical for our brain health. To make the best food choices, and the best fat choices, we must look at the major studies and decide for ourselves, in collaboration with our medical providers, what is best for our long-term health.

CHAPTER 8

# The Complexities of Carbohydrates

CARBOHYDRATES ARE A MIXED BLESSING. ON ONE HAND, THEY are an excellent source of glucose, nutrients, and fiber. On the other hand, they contribute to the epidemic of obesity attributed to our Western diet. How can one category of food have such a contrary effect on our health? The answer lies in the diversity and complexity of the carbohydrates themselves.

Carbohydrates are divided into two groups, simple and complex. When simple and complex carbohydrates are digested, they become primarily glucose, a major nutrient for the body. The simpler the carbohydrate, the more rapidly it breaks down and enters the bloodstream. The more complex the carbohydrate, the longer it takes to be broken down and absorbed into the blood. Simple carbs, sometimes labeled "bad" carbs, are small molecules that are immediately digested. If eaten alone without fats and proteins, simple carbohydrates cause the blood sugar to rise very quickly or peak. Complex carbohydrates, the "good" carbohydrates, are larger molecules and contain less sugar and more fiber, protein, and fat, so they take longer to digest. Because they enter the bloodstream more slowly, complex carbohydrates are a more constant and even source of energy.

Many processed foods are simple carbohydrates. Examples are

bread, pasta, cookies, cakes, candy, sodas, fruit juices, and many packaged breakfast cereals. Whole foods like grapefruit, kiwi, pears, oranges, watermelon, potatoes, and milk are also simple carbs but contain natural vitamins, minerals, and fiber. Because of their sugar content, they are also digested and absorbed quickly.

Complex carbohydrates are generally whole, unprocessed foods that are lower in sugar than simple carbohydrates and rich in vitamins, minerals, and fiber. Whole grains; vegetables such as broccoli and cauliflower; leafy greens such as spinach, kale, and chard; some fruits such as apples, plums, cherries, and strawberries; and avocados, asparagus, lentils, beans, and peas are examples of complex carbohydrates.

## Carbohydrates and Obesity

American dietary guidelines have historically recommended carbohydrates make up the majority of our food intake. The 1992 *Food Guide Pyramid* recommended 6 to 11 servings of bread, cereal, rice, and pasta per day, and 5 to 9 servings of fruit and vegetables. The total amount of carbohydrates equaled 20 servings per day, or 70% of calories consumed. The remaining recommendations were protein and dairy, up to six servings per day or 30% of the diet. The recommendations also say, "Fat, oils and sweets are to be used sparingly."

The revision of the *Food Guide Pyramid, MyPlate,* recommends 30% grains and 50% fruits and vegetables. The remaining recommended 20% is protein. The percentage of carbohydrates at 80% is even higher than the amount of carbohydrates recommended by the *Food Guide Pyramid.* Low-fat dairy is to the side, not included on the plate. There is no mention of fat except to warn that fried chicken, whole milk, cheese, and ground beef (25% fat) are empty calories. The 1977 *Dietary Goals for the United States* recommended we reduce our fat intake from 40% to 30%. In 2010 another 10% reduction was recommended. The current USDA recommendation of fat intake is just 20% of total calories consumed. Today nutritionists believe a healthy diet contains 40 to 60% fat.

With the recommendations to reduce fat consumption and increase carbohydrate consumption, it would seem Americans should be getting thinner rather than fatter. However, obesity rates have more than doubled in both adults and children since the 1970s. According to the Food Research and Action Center (FRAC), 68.8% of adults are now overweight or obese and 31.8% of children are overweight or obese. Researchers note that this is the first generation of children, because of their diet, who will not live longer than their parents.

How did Americans get so overweight? The emphasis on high carbohydrate intake recommended by the *Dietary Guidelines for Americans* and *MyPlate* has fueled the increase. It's also the kind of carbohydrates we're eating. The typical American diet is filled with processed foods, and many are made from the simple carbohydrates flour and sugar. Americans consume on average of 133 pounds of wheat per year, and more than 85% of the grains we eat are processed. Wheat increases blood sugar more than table sugar. Two hundred years ago Americans ate two pounds of sugar per year. Today we consume 152 pounds per year.

To understand why carbohydrates are responsible for weight gain, we need to know how the body processes them.

## Glucose Regulation

**Glucose and insulin.** Glucose, a form of sugar, is one of the nutrient end products of the digestive process and a major source of fuel for the body. Most of the carbohydrates we eat become glucose. The body's goal is to maintain a perfect level of glucose in the blood. Insulin, a hormone secreted in the pancreas gland, has the job of regulating glucose. A balanced meal of protein, fat, and complex carbohydrates will digest slowly. The glucose enters the bloodstream in a steady flow so our energy supply is constant. Any glucose not needed immediately is stored as glycogen in the skeletal muscles or in the liver. If there is excess glucose and the storage capacity of both the muscles and the liver is reached, glucose is stored as fat.

When our bodies need more energy between meals, the glycogen, stored glucose, is released from the muscles. If that supply is depleted, glycogen is released from the liver. The last source of energy to be burned is fat. However, if the insulin levels remain high because there is still glucose in the blood, the fat stored in our liver and tissues is not available. Carbohydrates stored as fat cannot be released while insulin is present. Over time, as we continue to eat more carbohydrates than we can burn, fat continues to be stored and unavailable. It accumulates throughout our bodies and we gain weight, and in extreme cases, become obese. In spite of all that we have been told, it is not the fat that we eat that causes us to get fat. It is the storage of carbohydrates as fat that cannot be retrieved and burned. To burn fat, carbohydrate intake must be curtailed. When less glucose is available, a process called ketosis begins. Ketosis is the burning of fat instead of glucose. That's the rationale behind a low carbohydrate diet often being suggested for weight loss.

**The team: glucagon and insulin.** Another important hormone, glucagon, also helps regulate blood sugar levels. Glucagon is secreted by the pancreas and works in collaboration with insulin. In-between meals, when blood sugar is depleted, glucagon is activated to release stored glycogen. Stored glycogen is pulled from tissues and the liver to raise blood sugar levels. When glycogen is depleted, fat will be released and burned. Ideally, insulin and glucagon work together: insulin to get the glucose out of the blood and into the tissues and liver, and glucagon to get glucose back into the blood from the tissues and liver or stored fat when blood sugar is low. These two hormones work in tandem to maintain our energy and keep blood sugar in balance.

**Leptin and hunger regulation.** Another hormone, leptin, also comes into play. Leptin is secreted primarily by the fat cells of the belly, buttocks, and thighs. Insulin, as it works to regulate blood sugar, activates the fat cell metabolism, producing leptin. Leptin travels from the fat cells to the brain to stop hunger messages when your stomach is full. Leptin also tells your pancreas to stop producing insulin because it's no longer needed.

When an adequate amount of food is consumed for your activity level, both insulin levels and leptin levels drop. However, with continuous overeating, consuming more calories than your body can burn, insulin remains in the blood and stimulates the production of triglycerides (fats). High concentrations of triglycerides prevent the leptin from reaching the brain. If this occurs over time, leptin resistance sets in and hunger is not regulated. The brain does not get the message to stop eating, and continued eating creates excess glucose. The excess glucose, now in the form of triglycerides, becomes fat and is stored. High triglycerides may raise the risk of heart disease.

Insulin, glucagon, and leptin work in a delicate, three-way dance, regulating not only blood sugar and energy production, but also appetite and fat storage.

**Carbohydrates and cholesterol.** High carbohydrate consumption also affects cholesterol levels. Seventy to eighty percent of cholesterol comes, not from food, but from the liver. One of the main functions of cholesterol is to provide the structural framework for all cells. Insulin and glucagon mediate this process. When there is too much insulin circulating in the blood, cholesterol-making enzymes are activated, stimulating the overproduction of cholesterol. The overproduction of cholesterol serves a purpose. It helps create new cells that are needed to store the fat we have been unable to burn because of the insulin present in the blood. It's an elegant and efficient process. A diet high in carbohydrates not only produces fat but also helps create the cells to store it. However, if carbohydrate intake is reduced, glucagon steps in and cholesterol-making enzymes are deactivated, reducing the amount of cholesterol produced, and cholesterol levels go down.

**Insulin resistance.** When the body is flooded with sugar and simple carbohydrates, insulin pours into the bloodstream to manage the glucose, causing insulin spikes. A small serving of sugary breakfast cereal that contains 15 grams of sugar will increase both the glucose and the insulin concentration. If this happens habitually, the finely tuned process that controls blood sugar levels is disrupted and creates a condition called insulin resistance. Insulin resistance develops when insulin receptor cells become insensitive or resistant to the insulin, requiring more insulin to circulate in the blood to regulate the blood sugar. Even though there is more insulin, the glucose lowering effects of insulin are reduced, leaving dangerously high levels of sugar in the blood. Insulin resistance is the beginning of a downward spiral that leads to unregulated blood sugar. A person with an ongoing, unregulated, abnormally high level of blood sugar may become a type 2 diabetic. Insulin resistance increases the risk for cancer and also sets in motion the formation of plaques that are present in the brains of people with Alzheimer's.

**Metabolic syndrome.** Metabolic syndrome is a condition of three or more related health problems that may have their origins in insulin resistance. The increased level of insulin pumped out by the pancreas to regulate blood sugar levels promotes fat storage, increases blood pressure, and elevates levels of cholesterol and triglycerides. The presence of so much blood sugar and insulin generates large numbers of hazardous free radicals and sets the stage for heart disease, cancer, Alzheimer's, and other diseases. Metabolic syndrome is diagnosed in the presence of three or more of these components: elevated waist circumference, elevated triglycerides, reduced HDL (good cholesterol), elevated blood pressure, and elevated fasting glucose levels.

**Glycation.** An extended period of high blood sugar also causes a harmful process called glycation, the bonding of amino acids, a form of protein, to sugar. The bonding of these two molecules, or advanced glycosylation end products (AGEs), causes oxidation stress and the production of free radicals. When this new form of molecule is taken into and used by body tissues, it damages arteries and affects the collagen of the skin, the muscles and tendons, the delicate lenses of the eyes, and the myelin sheaths around the nerves.

Glycation is a major cause of the aging process, including

memory loss. Aging is essentially the glycation of all tissue, including the brain. It causes aging of the skin because it disrupts the repair process of collagen fibers. It causes the myelin sheaths around the nerves to deteriorate and interferes with the regeneration of the nerve fibers. Because the brain is not particularly sensitive to insulin, it is more vulnerable to glycation and the oxidation and creation of free radicals that results in memory loss and cognitive decline. Glycation is implicated in Alzheimer's disease, cardiovascular disease, and diabetes. A dramatic piece of evidence of glycation is the damage found in people with advanced stages of diabetes who lose their limbs and eyesight.

## Carbohydrates and Your Brain

An estimated 110,000 Americans die as a result of obesity each year and about one-third of all cancers are directly related to it. Obesity is also linked to heart disease, type 2 diabetes, and stroke, but new research links obesity to brain degeneration as well. Obese persons are at increased risk for brain atrophy and dementia as they age.

Neurology scientists from the University of California in Los Angeles found that obese people have 8% less brain tissue than normal weight individuals, and their brains appear to have aged eight years prematurely. They had lost brain tissue in the frontal lobes, areas of the brain critical for planning and memory, and in the anterior cingulate gyrus (attention and executive functions), hippocampus (long-term memory), and basal ganglia (movement). Diabetes is a risk factor for dementia and these scientists' studies suggest that higher glucose levels may be a risk factor for dementia even among persons without diabetes.

Researchers tracked 1,230 people between the ages of 70 and 89 and found that those who reported consuming the highest amount of carbohydrates were 1.9 times more likely to develop mild cognitive impairment than those with the lowest intake. Incidence of mental decline was 1.5 times higher in people with the highest sugar intake compared to the lowest. Those who adhered to a diet high in "good fats" (nuts and healthy oils) were 42% less likely to experience cognitive impairment. People with a high intake of other forms of protein and fats (meat and fish) cut their risk by 21%.

Researchers concluded that people should eat a healthy balance of carbohydrates, fat, and protein to protect their brains, because once mild cognitive impairment starts, it is difficult to stop its progression.

## Why You Should Eat Your Veggies (and Fruits)

Two major categories of carbohydrates are fruits and vegetables. Vegetables are seldom on most people's lists of favorite foods, but our brains and bodies love them. Fruits fare better and we're more likely to eat them because they're sweet. The USDA's *MyPlate* recommends that half our plates be fruits and vegetables, and here they are right on. Plants contain thousands of natural chemicals called phytonutrients that may help prevent disease and promote health. Although these organic components are not "essential" for life, they are pro-health and pro-life. Many of the phytonutrients are also antioxidants and provide us with protection from free radicals that cause inflammation. Phytonutrients are just beginning to be understood and hundreds of studies are currently underway to explore the role they play in our overall health. Below are examples of several well-known phytonutrients, where they are found, and how they promote good health.

**Carotenoids.** This class of phytonutrients is found in yellow, orange, pink, and green fruits and vegetables. Examples are peaches, apricots, watermelon, pink grapefruit, tomatoes, carrots, yellow squash, pumpkins, broccoli, and green leafy vegetables such as kale, spinach, and collard greens. Carotenoids act as antioxidants and fight free radicals that damage tissues throughout the body.

**Flavonoids.** Virtually all fruits and vegetables contain flavonoids. As an antioxidant, they are one of the most healthful and helpful phytonutrients. Flavonoids have many functions, including protecting cell structures, preventing excessive inflammation, and acting as an antibiotic by disrupting the function of viruses and bacteria.

**Resveratrol.** Resveratrol has received much attention lately because of its presence in wine and dark red grapes. It acts as an antioxidant and anti-inflammatory. Recent research also suggests it may have anti-aging properties, because it mimics calorie restriction in some ways and has extended the lifespans of yeast, worms, flies, and fish. It appears to increase the activity of the mitochondria, the organelles that product the cell's energy.

**Ellagic acid.** Ellagic acid may have some anti-cancer properties. Laboratory studies have found that it may cause cell death in cancer cells, reduce the effect of estrogen in promoting growth of breast cancer cells, and help the liver break down or remove some cancer-causing substances in the blood. Studies are still underway to determine if ellagic acid can prevent or treat cancer in humans. It is found in strawberries, raspberries, and pomegranates, particularly if they are freeze-dried; and in walnuts, cranberries, pecans, and other plant foods.

**Glucosinolates.** Cruciferous vegetables such as broccoli, cabbage, kale, and Brussels sprouts get their sharp odor and flavor from the glucosinolates within the plant. Eating ample amounts of these vegetables is associated with a reduced risk of cancer, particularly lung cancer and cancers of the gastrointestinal tract.

## The Problem with Grains

Although grains have been around for thousands of years and have provided a reliable source of nutrients, they come with baggage. Studies looking at fossil records and Egyptian mummies concluded that as Egyptians relied more on agricultural products, as farming replaced hunting and gathering, and grains replaced lean meat, fish, vegetables, nuts, seeds, and fruits, many of the diseases we know today became common. Heart disease, obesity, bone diseases such as osteoporosis, tooth decay, dental diseases, arthritis, obesity, infectious diseases, and birth defects were found in greater numbers. Adding insult to injury, Egyptians did not live as long as their hunter/gatherer forerunners.

Current research on grains is inconclusive. Epidemiological studies, those studies involving huge populations combining a number of other smaller studies, show an association between diets high in whole grains and lower C-reactive protein (CRP) concentrations. CRP is a marker for inflammation throughout the body. On the other hand, interventional studies, those that involve some kind change in practice, do not demonstrate a clear effect of increased whole grain consumption on CRP or other markers of inflammation. The type of whole grain in these studies is not defined, so the outcomes are ambiguous. Many whole grains contain gluten, which creates inflammation for those who are sensitive or allergic to grain. The studies do not specifically address celiac disease or gluten sensitivity.

The benefits of whole grain have been described as reducing systemic inflammation and protecting against both type 2 diabetes and cardiovascular disease. They also provide a good source of fiber. Research has linked high fiber intake to lower levels of inflammation. However, it is clear that consuming whole grains and refined or processed grains produces different outcomes.

Eating whole grains may prevent weight gain and therefore reduce the amount of inflammation in the body caused by obesity and related disorders. Whole grains also contain bran, endosperm, and the germ of the plant and retain the beneficial vitamins, minerals, and fiber that are lost in processed grains.

High intake of refined grains, on the other hand, boosts levels of inflammatory proteins. Processed grains are devoid of fiber, minerals, vitamins, and fatty acids, and their consumption spikes glucose levels, increasing the need for insulin. Many cereals are "fortified" to replace the nutrients removed in their processing.

Cereal grains, a major source of food in our Western diet, are poor sources of calcium, vitamin C, vitamin A, and except for yellow corn, beta-carotene. If eaten to excess, grain calcium can displace more beneficial dairy and vegetable calcium, and can negatively impact bone growth and metabolism by limiting calcium absorption and by altering vitamin D metabolism. Pellagra and beriberi, two B vitamin deficiency diseases, are almost exclusively associated with excessive grain consumption. B6, which performs over one hundred functions in the body, is less easily absorbed from cereal grains than from animal products. Grain consumption also elevates blood glucose levels and triggers cravings for sweets. Gluten and a high carbohydrate diet are among the most potent stimulators of inflammation to the brain.

**Celiac disease and gluten sensitivity.** Food biologists have been breeding hybrid grains that produce more yield per acre, a bigger grain head, and a shorter stock for decades. Over time, the quality of the grain has been altered so it scarcely resembles the grain of our grandparents'. One of the major changes has been the increase in gluten in the grain. Gluten is the protein found in wheat, barley, and rye, and its presence has led to an epidemic of celiac disease. Celiac disease is an autoimmune disorder that triggers body-wide inflammation.

Gluten damages the gut lining of people with celiac disease, allowing partially digested food to leak across the gut barrier, activating the immune system in the gut. Symptoms of celiac disease include irritable bowel-like symptoms, joint or bone pain, headaches, fatigue and weakness, depression, irritability, mood disorders, swelling and inflammation, low blood sugar, headaches, fatigue, bloating, gas, constipation, diarrhea, eczema, weight loss or weight gain, and in some cases, malnourishment. When people diagnosed with celiac disease, they must eat a gluten free diet for the remainder of their lives. Deviation from the diet can reactive their symptoms. Celiac disease affects 1 in 100 people in the United States.

New research indicates that not only does gluten cause celiac disease, creating serious digestive problems, it also affects brain tissue. Non-celiac gluten sensitivity may occur independently of celiac and is not associated with celiac disease or gut damage. Gluten sensitivity primarily attacks the brain and the nervous system and may damage those areas more than any other tissue in the body. Here's how it works. The immune system may mistake nerve cell protein for gluten protein and create antibodies to fight against the gluten protein, but because they are so similar, the antibodies also destroy the nervous system protein. Because of this mistaken identity, gluten sensitivity can cause vascular damage and a number of neurological problems. Some scientists believe many neurological problems are caused by inflammation and they identify gluten sensitivity as a primary cause of the inflammation.

Two factors contribute to the increase in both celiac and gluten sensitivity. The first is the on-going hybridization of wheat. Hybridization creates new protein by combining different strains of wheat, altering the protein sequence of the grain, and changing its original form. The new proteins appear to trigger an immune response, particularly in the brain and nervous system.

Secondly, a process called deamidation, used in food processing, employs acids or enzymes to make gluten soluble so it mixes more readily with other foods. Deamidation creates a new food compound that has been shown to cause a severe immune response in people with gluten sensitivity.

Non-celiac gluten sensitivity is on the rise. An estimated 30 to 40% of the world's population may have the gene for susceptibility. Some symptoms are the same as celiac disease but lack the severity of the actual gluten intolerance. Although it is believed to be widespread, many medical practitioners are reluctant to diagnose gluten sensitivity because it has such a variety of symptoms. One way to determine if you have gluten intolerance is to eliminate gluten for two weeks to see if your symptoms subside. However, there are foods that contain proteins that are so similar to gluten that your body confuses them for gluten, a condition called cross reactivity.

Some of those foods are soy, yeast, chocolate, eggs, millet, coffee, corn, and a dozen others.

The following are gluten-containing grains and gluten-free grains. (Whole Grains Council)

| Grains with Gluten | | Gluten-Free Grains | |
|---|---|---|---|
| Wheat | Durum | Buckwheat | Sorghum |
| Spelt | Kamut | Corn* | Wild rice |
| Bulgur | Semolina | Millet | Rice |
| Barley | Farro | Quinoa | Amaranth |
| Rye | | Teff | Oats** |

\* Corn contains several glutens, unrelated to wheat gluten, that may cause atrophy to intestinal villi.

\*\* Oats are essentially gluten-free but may be contaminated with wheat during growing or processing.

According to the author of *Wheat Belly*, Dr. William Davis, wheat contains compounds that not only cause inflammatory responses, such as celiac disease and gluten sensitivity, it contains compounds that are also highly addictive. One of the byproducts of digested wheat is exorphin, a morphine-like compound that binds to opiate receptors in the brain. The result is appetite stimulation and addictive behavior. Dr. Davis suggests that exorphin can result in the consumption of more than 400 additional calories per day.

The alternatives to wheat, kamut and spelt, also produce exorphin through digestion, although not in the same amount as wheat. Kamut and spelt still contain gluten and lectins. Other common grains, such as rice, oats, and corn, are high in carbohydrates and increase blood sugar. Buckwheat, quinoa, millet, and amaranth are technically seeds but still raise blood sugar. They also inhibit the absorption of many minerals, including calcium, magnesium, iron, and zinc, among others. Millet is particularly problematic because it hinders the uptake of iodine, suppressing thyroid functioning. Corn contains several glutens and appears to cause the villi of the intestines to atrophy. GMO corn is also implicated in damage and inflammation of intestinal cells.

**Lectin.** Lectin, another protein found in plants, is implicated in inflammation as well. Lectins are an important part of the plant's natural immune system and provide a protective barrier for the plant from invaders such as plant eaters, mold, or parasites. They also keep the plant from germinating until the proper conditions are present. Your body is unable to digest or destroy the lectin proteins because they are resistant to breakdown in the stomach or intestines. They can penetrate the mucus membrane of the intestines and become deposited in the internal organs. Lectins can attach to various cells, such as the endothelial cells in the brain. The immune system sees the lectin as a foreign invader and attack, altering the structure, function, and communication of cells. Many food allergies are actually the immune system's reaction to lectins.

Lectins are found in many of the foods we eat. Nightshade plants such as tomatoes, potatoes, and eggplants; all milk products, including cheese and yogurt; legumes; eggs; and all beans, including soy and peanuts, contain some quantities of lectins. Your susceptibility to lectins depends on your individual genetic code. Almost everyone has antibodies to some dietary lectins in their bloodstream.

**Enzyme inhibitors, phytic acid, and other issues.** A wide variety of foods are important for maintaining a balanced diet, but some foods can have unexpected components. Grains, legumes, and tubers contain enzyme inhibitors and phytic acid. They exist on the plant, similar to lectins, as a coating that protects their seeds (grains, legumes, and tubers are seeds) from predators and prevents premature germination. The coatings of the seeds are noxious to animals, worms, and insects and are natural pesticides that guard against bacteria and other life forms that may threaten the plants. However, the enzyme inhibitors prevent our digestive enzymes from breaking down the food. The phytic acid combines with iron, calcium, magnesium, copper, and zinc in the intestinal tract and blocks their absorption.

Examples of amounts of phytic acid in some popular grain products include: oatmeal: 943 milligrams/100 grams, and wheat bran:

3,011 milligrams/100 grams. Vegetables by comparison are very low in phytic acid. An avocado contains 1 milligram/100 grams and broccoli 18 milligrams/100 grams.

## Preparing Grains, Legumes, and Tubers

Indigenous societies that use grain, legumes, or tubers as their main food sources usually soak or ferment their foods before consuming them. The processes neutralize phytic acid and enzyme inhibitors in grain and help break down the complex sugars in legumes. Contemporary societies process their food in similar ways. The Japanese ferment soybeans to produce miso and coagulate soymilk to produce tofu. Mexicans soak beans, and soak and mash corn before cooking. South Americans ferment cassava before grinding it into flour. In Europe and America wheat is fermented to produce sour dough bread.

Sprouting, soaking overnight, or fermenting acts as a predigestion process that allows many people who otherwise could not tolerate these foods to digest them. Not only do these processes help neutralize the phytic acid and enzyme inhibitors, they also improve the nutritional value by increasing the production of numerous beneficial enzymes and the amounts of vitamins, particularly B vitamins, and make the proteins more available for absorption.

## Fiber

Fiber, a component of carbohydrates, is part of the plant that is not digestible. Instead of being absorbed by the body, fiber passes through the stomach, small intestine, colon, and out as stool. Fiber is necessary for good digestion. There are two kinds of fiber, soluble and insoluble, although many plants contain some of each.

**Soluble fiber.** Soluble fiber dissolves in water and forms a gel-like material that slows down digestion. It delays the emptying of your stomach so you feel full longer, helping to maintain a healthy weight. Because it slows digestion, it helps stabilize blood sugar levels. Fiber also helps lower LDL ("bad") cholesterol by interfering with the absorption of dietary cholesterol. Examples of foods with soluble fiber include citrus fruits, pears, peas, strawberries, blueberries, oatmeal, lentils, cucumbers, celery, and carrots.

**Insoluble fiber.** Insoluble fiber does not dissolve in water, so it passes through the gastrointestinal tract relatively intact. Insoluble fiber has a laxative effect and speeds up the passage of food through the gut and helps prevent constipation. It also helps soften and increase the size of the stool. Foods that contain insoluble fiber include whole grains and vegetables, including beets, potatoes, and other root vegetables with their skins.

**Recommended fiber intake.** The American Heart Association recommends 14 grams of fiber for every 1,000 calories eaten, or as a general recommendation, 25 grams of fiber per day. It does not distinguish between soluble and insoluble fiber. Studies indicate that Americans do not eat half the fiber recommended.

**Health benefits of fiber.** A high fiber diet causes food to pass through the digestive system quickly, which scientists believe protects against some cancers. High fiber intake may also reduce the risk of hemorrhoids and diverticular disease. Several new studies show that adequate fiber intake may also reduce the risk of heart disease and stroke.

The *Journal of American College of Cardiology* reported a study that followed 39,876 women for six years and found that those who ingested an average of 26.3 grams of fiber daily were at lower risk of developing heart disease or having a heart attack than those who ate less. The American Heart Association journal *Stroke* reported that eating more fiber was linked to a lower risk for first time stroke. Every seven-gram increase in total dietary fiber was associated with a seven percent lower risk of first time stroke. Eating dietary fiber is particularly important for people who have stroke risk factors, such as age, obesity, high blood pressure, or smoking. Stroke is the fourth leading cause of death in the US, and among survivors, the leading cause of disability.

# Rethink Your Carbohydrate Intake

Carbohydrates are a perfect example of too much of a good thing. As an important source of nutrients and fiber, they need to be consumed with discretion. Simple carbohydrates can upset the delicate balance of blood sugar; complex carbohydrates give us a more constant source of energy but have unintended consequences. Grains, the darling of the *Food Guide Pyramid* and *MyPlate*, can cause obesity and inflammation, leading to many of the modern, preventable diseases. Grains, seeds, and tubers need to be processed, not as our industrial food producers do, but as indigenous people do, through soaking, mashing, and fermenting. Carbohydrates, prepared as our ancestors ate them, will provide the most digestible, non-inflammatory nutrients.

CHAPTER 9

# Protein: The Building Blocks

B ESIDES WATER, PROTEIN IS THE MOST ABUNDANT MOLECULE IN our bodies. It's the major structural component of every living cell. Hair, nails, and outer layers of skin are made of protein. Muscles contain a variety of proteins. Organs are made of it and so are bones. Red blood cells contain hemoglobin, a protein compound that carries oxygen throughout the body. Blood plasma is made of lipoproteins and transports fat and proteins. Enzymes, made of proteins, have specific tasks, such as digesting food and making new cells. Chromosomes, made up of nucleoproteins, have components of protein in them. The brain depends on proteins to build its neurotransmitters to support its communication network and to maintain memory. Without an adequate amount of protein, the body would waste away and the brain could not function.

## Proteins Are Amino Acids

Protein is one of the three macronutrients needed by the body, along with fat and carbohydrates. Proteins are a polymer chain made of amino acids linked together by peptide bonds. During digestion, proteins are broken down into single amino acids. Each amino acid has a specific function. Amino acids are divided into three categories: essential amino acids, nonessential amino acids, and conditional amino acids. The category refers to whether or not they can be made by the body. Essential amino acids cannot be made or stored, so we must get them from food. During digestion, the body makes nonessential amino acids from essential amino acids. Conditional amino acids are not essential unless a person is sick, stressed, or has a serious long-term illness.

There are nine essential amino acids, four nonessential amino acids, and eight conditional amino acids. The essential amino acids are histidine, isoleucine, leucine, lysine, methionine, phenylalanine, threonine, tryptophan, and valine. The nonessential amino acids are alanine, aspartic acid, glutamic acid, and selenocysteine. The conditional amino acids are arginine, cysteine, glutamine, tyrosine, glycine, ornithine, proline, and serine.

Meat, poultry, fish, dairy, and eggs are complete proteins containing all the amino acids. Incomplete proteins must be combined to insure all necessary amino acids are present. The pairing of rice and beans is an example. The best sources of plant protein comes from legumes, such as lentils, kidney beans, white beans, chickpeas, and tofu, and from nuts and seeds, such as Brazil nuts, cashews, pecans, and sunflower and sesame seeds. Sixty percent of the world's population exists on incomplete proteins, because they are cheaper and more readily available. North Americas consume 70% of their protein from animals.

## Why Proteins Are Important

Protein digests more slowly than carbohydrates and thus tempers the rise in blood sugar. Protein helps maintain a feeling of satiation, curbing hunger for longer periods of time than carbohydrates. Although it's primary function is building and maintenance, it can be burned as a fuel like carbohydrates and fat when supplies of carbohydrates and fats are low.

Proteins help regulate appetite. In the journal article "Brain Response to High-Protein Diets," the authors explain that they found that eating protein sends signals from the gut to the brain, via the vagus nerve, to stop eating when a sufficient quantity of protein has been consumed. The information led to new approaches to dieting for persons who are obese or overweight. Higher levels of protein intake, when compared with average protein intake, seem to provide good long-term maintenance of reduced visceral fat and, when combined with exercise, lean mass gain.

In normal circumstances, physical activity and exertion increase the need for protein. Competitive athletes have a greater need for protein than sedentary adults. Growing children, adolescents, and nursing mothers also need more protein. A lack of protein will cause the body to burn muscle mass to provide energy, and in extreme cases of a severe diet or starvation, the muscles can be partially consumed. Lack of protein can also cause failure to thrive, increased susceptibility to disease, weakening of the heart and respiratory systems, brain dysfunction, and even death.

Ideally, protein supplies 25% of adult energy requirements. This translates into 46 grams per day for sedentary adult women 19 to 70 years of age and 56 grams for sedentary adult men 19 to 70 years of age. Another way to calculate need is to consume about 8 grams of protein for every 20 pounds of body weight. Very active people will need to consume more. Visually, one-fourth of your food plate should be a protein. Here are examples of amounts of protein in food:

- Hamburger patty, 4 ounces—28 grams
- Chicken breast, 3.5 ounces—30 grams
- Tuna, 6-ounce can—40 grams
- Pork tenderloin, 4 ounces—29 grams
- Egg, large—6 grams
- Most beans, ½ cup cooked,—7–10 grams
- Almonds, ¼ cup—8 grams

# Proteins and Brain Function

Proteins are an integral part of brain structure and brain function. The amino acids within the proteins are the building blocks of the brain's network. Beef, fish, chicken, and eggs each contain twenty-two amino acids.

Proteins provide material for creating cell structure and the growth of the long axons that extend from nerve cell bodies. They carry glucose, the primary fuel for the brain, from the blood to the brain through the blood brain barrier. Proteins supply the amino acids that regulate the brain's chemical and electrical activity through the neurotransmitters, hormones, and enzymes. Amino acids regulate both appetite and mood. Protein is essential for healthy brain functioning.

# Choose Proteins Carefully

Although animal products are the best source of complete proteins, they are not free of controversy. Factory farms raise both ethical and nutritional issues, calling into question the large-scale production of cattle, hogs, chickens, and fish. Red meat containing saturated fat has been implicated in the development of heart disease. Beans and legumes also have their issues. As Chapter 6 explains, vegetable protein, if not prepared properly, can cause inflammation and leaky gut, which lead to chronic diseases. What shall we eat?

**The red meat controversy.** For years the saturated fat in red meat was believed to be the cause of high cholesterol and heart disease, in spite of compelling evidence to the contrary. The red meat controversy was stoked by an April 2013 article published in the journal *Nature Medicine*. The authors wrote that the intestinal microbiota metabolism of L-carnitine, a nutrient in red meat, produces a byproduct called trimethylamine N-oxide (TMAO), which promotes heart disease. The popular press jumped on the study and headlines read, "Eating Red Meat Increases Death Risk." But the study has been highly criticized. Many scientists found the research methods of the authors questionable and their conclusions controversial. Other researchers point out that many foods, including fruits and vegetables, also produce TMOA.

An earlier article (2010) that included over 1.2 million participants found no correlation between the consumption of fresh, unprocessed red meat and the increased risk of heart disease, stroke, or diabetes. However, the consumption of processed meat was associated with a 42% higher risk of heart disease and a 19% higher risk for diabetes. The association with stroke was not conclusive. For studies on the lack of correlation between heart disease and saturated fat see Chapter 7.

**Factory farms.** Most animal proteins available in supermarkets are raised on large farms called combined animal feeding operations (CAFOs), or factory farms. Beef cattle, dairy cows, hogs, poultry, sheep, goats, and fish are raised under conditions that disregard their natural behavior and their natural food. Most are confined in small, crowded spaces and fed hormones to accelerate their growth and antibiotics to compensate for the diseases that flourish in the deplorable conditions. Humane conditions are sacrificed for corporate profit.

Over nine billion animals are raised and slaughtered on factory farms each year. For the amount of meat they produce, they use huge quantities of natural resources and produce enormous quantities of waste and greenhouse gases. Producing one pound of beef takes an estimated 1,581 gallons of water. Animals raised on factory farms in the US generate more than one million pounds of manure per day.

The Environmental Protection Agency estimates that between 1990 and 2005, methane emissions from hog and cow operations rose 37% and 50% respectively, due largely to the greater amount and concentration of manure in lagoons and related storage systems. This huge amount of animal waste contributes to greenhouse gases. One specific kind of animal waste byproduct associated with hog production also yields hydrogen sulfide, which can cause neurological and cardiac disorders, seizures, and psychological problems.

Upwards of 70% of the antibiotics produced in this country are fed to animals for non-therapeutic purposes. While the goal is to prevent the livestock from becoming sick from their food and environment, the excessive use of the medication contributes to antibiotic resistant bacteria in humans. Furthermore, the growth hormones given to dairy cows to promote growth and increase milk production have been shown to significantly increase the risk of breast, prostate, and colon cancers in humans. The hormones are also believed to be contributing to the early sexual development of children.

A series of studies from prestigious universities, published in peer-reviewed scientific journals, demonstrates just how bizarre our food production has become. Researchers discovered that arsenic is being fed to chickens and hogs to reduce infections and to color their flesh pink. Chickens were also given an antihistamine, the active ingredient in Benadryl. In some studies, acetaminophen, the active ingredient in Tylenol, and the antidepressant found in Prozac were also found. While using tranquilizers to calm them down, the chickens were fed coffee pulp and green tea to keep them awake so they would eat for longer hours. Researcher also found banned antibiotics.

**Dairy as a protein source.** If we are lucky, we begin life drinking mother's milk, the perfect food for an infant. It comes with the right mix of fat, protein, and carbohydrates. Unfortunately, as we grow older and substitute cow's milk for mother's milk, it's not so perfect. Many adults have problems consuming dairy products, because they no longer produce the enzyme lactose, which is necessary for digesting milk. Others are allergic to the milk protein casein, one of the most difficult proteins for the body to digest.

For people who are able to tolerate milk, they have a choice between raw milk or processed (pasteurized and homogenized) milk and organic or non-organic milk. Raw, full-fat milk from pasture-fed cows contains vital nutrients, such as fat-soluble vitamins A and D, calcium, conjugated linoleic acid (CLA), and vitamins B6 and B12. Raw milk is a complete protein that contains beneficial bacteria that protects against pathogens and contributes to a healthy gut environment. Butterfat contains short- and medium-chain acids and glycosphingolipids that stimulate the immune system and prevent intestinal distress. Culturing raw milk enhances its probiotic and enzyme content, improving digestive health.

It is difficult to find raw milk in most states, unless it's purchased directly from a farmer. However, just recently, the FDA reversed its position, and it's no longer illegal to transport raw milk across state lines. Raw milk is much more available in Europe, where it is distributed under closely monitored conditions.

Organic whole milk is more nutritious than nonorganic whole milk. A recent study (2013) by scientists at the University of Washington compared whole pasteurized organic milk to whole pasteurized nonorganic milk. They found the organic milk contained 62% more omega-3 fatty acids and 25% less omega-6 fatty acids than conventional milk. Historically, saturated fat in milk and other dairy products has been linked to cardiovascular disease. On the other hand, consumption of full-fat dairy products has been linked to reduced incidences of cardiovascular disease, reduced weight gain, reduced markers for metabolic syndrome, and reduced colorectal cancer.

Current recommendations by the USDA suggest limiting full-fat dairy products in favor of low-fat or non-fat products. A conference statement published in the *European Journal of Nutrition*, investigating the potential effects of dairy products on cardiovascular disease risk, concluded there was no clear evidence dairy food consumption was associated with a higher risk of cardiovascular disease. They stated, "Thus, recommendations to reduce dairy food consumption irrespective of the nature of the dairy product should be made with caution." A recent *Time* magazine article, from June 23, 2014, reported on a study that found the saturated fat in dairy products might be more protective of cardiovascular disease than the fats found in meat.

In *The Journal of the American Medical Association Pediatrics*, contributing authors Ludwig and Willett concluded that people, particularly children, who consume reduced-fat milk may eat more carbohydrates to feel satiated.

An alternative to cow milk is goat milk. Goat milk is a complete food in itself, containing vitamins, minerals, trace elements, electrolytes, enzymes, protein, and fatty acids. It is much easier to digest and contains more omega-3s than cow's milk. However, it is not readily available in supermarkets and most often must be purchased directly from farmers.

**Soy and soy products.** The World's Healthiest Foods website has placed soy foods on their "10 Most Controversial WHFoods List." Here is another protein that presents a variety of concerns. At the heart of the issue is the natural product versus the industrial, processed product. The research shows very different results for whole soybeans and naturally fermented soybean food.

Soy has been a dietary staple in the Asian diet for thousands of years. Initially, it may have been used as a cover crop to introduce nitrogen back into the soil. Around 500 BC, China developed fermentation techniques that made the soybeans more palatable and digestible. Its use as food quickly spread to other Asian countries. Tempeh, miso, fermented tofu, nattō, and tamari soy sauce were all popular forms of fermented soy. These food products were introduced in the United States around the 1800s.

In Asia, soy is used as a condiment. In the US it is most often used as a replacement for animal protein. Fermented soy foods are a healthy addition to the diet. However, most modern soy foods, rather than being fermented, are processed. Highly processed soy protein "isolates," "concentrates," and similarly refined soy products contain trypsin inhibitors that inhibit protein digestion and affect pancreatic function. They denature proteins, increase levels of carcinogens, and cause deficiencies in calcium and vitamin D. Particular concern is centered around extremely high levels of estrogen compounds found in babies who are fed soy-based formula. The mega doses of phytoestrogens in soy formula have been implicated in the premature sexual development of girls and the delayed or retarded sexual development in boys. Soy isolates have not been granted FDA GRAS (generally recognized as safe) status because of concerns regarding the presence of toxins and carcinogens in the processed product.

The Midwestern part of the United States now produces half the world's supply of soybeans. Ninety-nine percent of those soybeans are grown from genetically modified seeds. Soybeans have the highest contamination of pesticides of any of our foodstuffs. GMO products have not been fully studied for their impact on human health, but emerging information calls into question their long-term health benefits.

## Protein and Vegetarians

Vegetarians eliminate animal protein from their diets for philosophical or health reasons. Instead, they get their proteins from plant sources, such as various beans and soy, products like tofu, veggie burgers, soymilk, and nuts and seeds. Generally, their diets include less protein than meat eaters, but with an adequate calorie intake and a balanced plant based diet, they may be as healthy as meat eaters. However, poorly planned diets may be low in calcium, omega-3 fatty acids, vitamin D, iron, zinc, vitamin B2, and iodine. Vitamin B12 is the most common deficiency, because animal products are its primary source.

Several studies have documented the prevalence of B12 deficiency in vegans and vegetarians. A literature review by researchers from the East Carolina University found reported deficiency rates for specific populations of vegetarians. The deficiency rates of B12 were 62% among pregnant women; between 25 and 86% among children; between 21 and 41% among adolescents; and between 11 and 90% among the elderly. Another study tracking 174 apparently healthy people reported that 92% of the vegans had vitamin B12 deficiency. People who included milk and eggs were also deficient. Vitamin B12 can be obtained from supplements.

There are serious health concerns with vitamin B12 deficiencies. Deficiencies can lead to anemia, fatigue, weakness, nausea, and constipation. Long-term deficiencies can result in nerve changes, such as numbness, balance, memory problems, tingling in the hands and feet, and depression. The lack of vitamin B12 can boost blood levels of the amino acid homocysteine. High homocysteine levels can promote blockages in arteries over time, leading to heart disease and stroke.

An alternative perspective of vegetarianism was reported in the 2010 version of *Dietary Guidelines for Americans*. The report states:

> In prospective studies of adults, compared to non-vegetarian eating patterns, vegetarian-style eating patterns have been associated with improved health outcomes—lower levels of obesity, a reduced risk of cardiovascular disease, and lower total mortality. Several clinical trials have documented that vegetarian eating patterns lower blood pressure.
>
> On average, vegetarians consume a lower proportion of calories from fat (particularly saturated fatty acids); fewer overall calories; and more fiber, potassium, and vitamin C than do non-vegetarians. Vegetarians generally have a lower body mass index. These characteristics and other lifestyle factors associated with a vegetarian diet may contribute to the positive health outcomes that have been identified among vegetarians.

What accounts for the difference in outcomes for these studies? Vegetarian and vegans are generally more health conscious than the general population. Consumers who shop at health food stores, vegetarians and non-vegetarians alike, generally have better overall health than people who buy their food at regular markets. There may be confounding variables, like smoking and sedentary lifestyles, not taken into consideration.

## Change is Coming

There is a robust movement in food production toward pasture-raised and free-range animals and poultry. Educated and concerned consumers are demanding better quality protein, as well as more humane conditions for the animals and poultry. Full-fat, unprocessed milk, both cow and goat, is increasingly available. There is a growing movement back to small farms where the production methods can be managed without sacrificing either the quality of the product or the environment. However, it comes at a cost. Organic and naturally raised meat and poultry products are often more expensive and less available. Consumers vote with their purses, and as the demand for better products increases, availability and affordability may improve. In the current political environment, reducing the amount of animal protein we consume may be the best alternative, for both our health and the environment.

CHAPTER 10

# Beware: Sugar and Sugar Substitutes

THE AMERICAN DIET IS DAMAGING OUR HEALTH AND SUGAR IS one of the major culprits. Although we each have responsibility for our behavior, factors outside ourselves have insidiously influenced our eating patterns. The ubiquitous advertisement of soft drinks and the processing of super palatable foods, including sugary cereals, cinnamon rolls, pancakes, candies, cakes, cookies, specialty breads, unlimited flavors of ice cream, etc., have moved us away from real food. Processed, convenient foods are quick and easy and support our busy lifestyles.

The federal government has aided our unhealthy food choices. As part of its mandate "to provide general and comprehensive information to citizens" the USDA has long been discrediting fat. The current recommendation of consuming only 20% fat for our daily intake of calories has spawned a "fat-free/reduced-fat" industry. Without fat, food not only tastes like cardboard, it feels like cardboard in our mouths. It's flat and unsatisfying. To improve the taste and palatability of reduced-fat food, sugar is added. At the same time, the USDA is subsidizing the grain industry, particularly corn, so that high fructose corn syrup, the sweetener used in much of the processed food, is inexpensive and widely available.

Sugar, a simple carbohydrate, is now in almost everything we eat, from yogurt, soups, peanut butter, bacon, ketchup, salad dressings, cereals, to most baked goods, including bread. And sugar is addictive. According to brain scans, sugar lights up the pleasure centers of our brains like cocaine, and it is equally addictive. The more sugar we eat, the more sugar we crave. On average, we consume more than a third of a pound of sugar each day. That's 500 calories of sugar daily. The largest percentage of those calories comes from sugary soft drinks. Cane and beet sugars, candies, and baked goods, like cake and cookies, come next.

Consuming excess amounts of sugar, such as a 12 ounce can of cola containing 33 grams of sugar, causes the pancreas to release a spike of insulin. Insulin spikes are one of the main causes of inflammation, a precursor to most major diseases. Research documents that sugar contributes to diabetes, heart disease, cancer, atherosclerosis, decreased HDL, increased triglycerides, dementia, and Alzheimer's. It harms the arteries and nerves. Many cancers, particularly colon and breast cancers, feed on glucose, which promotes the cancer's growth.

## Sugar Promotes Diseases

**Diabetes.** According to the Center for Disease Control, 25.8 million people, children and adults, a total of 8.3% of the US population, have diabetes. If this trend continues, a third of the US adults could have diabetes by 2050. According to the World Health Organization (WHO) 346 million people worldwide—5% of all humans—will have diabetes by 2050.

In a healthy person, insulin produced by the pancreas binds to receptors on cells throughout the body, signaling the cells to absorb glucose for the bloodstream. In diabetes, the insulin is not present or is not functioning properly. There are two types of diabetes. Type 1, usually diagnosed in children, is an autoimmune disease that destroys the pancreatic cells that produce insulin. Instead of being used by the muscles, the sugars build up in the blood, creating a toxic combination that, over years, damages blood vessels, nerves, and organs, such as the kidneys and eyes. To prevent this from happening, people with type 1 diabetes must inject insulin to survive.

In type 2 diabetes, the cells are unable to use the insulin the pancreas is producing. Because the cells are unable to absorb the glucose, it continues to circulate in the blood, similarly to type 1 diabetes. As the glucose continues to circulate in the blood, it is not available to be used by the muscles and organs. Over time, too much glucose in the blood causes inflammation and serious damage to the eyes, kidneys, and nerves. In severe cases, blindness results or limbs may need to be amputated. Diabetes also contributes to heart disease and stroke.

There are consequences for the brain as well. Japanese researchers examined 1,000 men and women over the age of 60 and found that people with diabetes were twice as likely as other study participants to develop Alzheimer's in 15 years. Another study published by *The New England Journal of Medicine* found that above normal blood sugar, even in people without diabetes, is associated with an increased risk of dementia. The researchers discovered that any incremental increase in blood sugar was associated with an increased risk of dementia, and the higher the blood sugar, the higher the risk. They suspect that the inability of the brain to properly use glucose might be the key factor in the development of Alzheimer's.

**High fructose corn syrup and inflammation.** Fructose is a natural ingredient in many fruits and vegetables. It adds flavor and satisfies our evolutionary craving for sweetness. However, as a food additive, fructose is derived from sugar cane, sugar beets, and corn. High fructose corn syrup (HFCS) comes from corn syrup that has been processed by enzymes to change some of its glucose into fructose.

Since the 1970s, HFCS has been used commercially in soft drinks and baked goods, and it is in almost all processed foods. HFCS is very inexpensive to produce as a result of government subsidies for corn. It is also relatively inexpensive because of its high degree of sweetness, so less product provides more sweetness. HFCS also enhances the sweetness of other sugars. It is highly soluble, so it's easy to use. One of its primary benefits is its retention of moisture for long periods of time, allowing products to have a long shelf life, a characteristic highly desirable for processed foods.

High fructose corn syrup is an extremely potent inflammatory agent, damaging cells throughout the body. For example, one hundred calories of glucose (from a potato or bread or other starch) and 100 calories of table sugar (half glucose and half fructose) are metabolized differently and have different effects on the body. The calories are the same, but the metabolic consequences, because the sugar is half fructose, are quite different. The fructose component of sugar and HFCS is metabolized primarily by the liver, where it's converted to free fatty acids. The fatty acids are stored as fat cells around the heart, liver, and digestive organs. When fructose is consumed in large quantities or in combination with omega-6 polyunsaturated fats, it creates a blood lipid profile that is associated with a high risk for cardiovascular disease.

The digestion of fructose also creates endotoxins that lead to endotoxemia. Endotoxemia causes metabolic syndrome, fatty liver disease, and systemic inflammation. Metabolic disease is a cluster of symptoms that lead to cardiovascular disease, diabetes, and stroke. Fatty liver is the accumulation of fat in the liver that causes inflammation and scarring of the liver. Systemic inflammation is believed to be the underlying cause of most diseases. Fructose also promotes fat accumulation in adipose tissue, leading to obesity, and is closely associated with many other diseases, including diabetes.

Another byproduct of fructose digestion is the creation of uric acid, which accumulates in the joints, causing a painful condition called gout. Fructose also increases your insulin and leptin levels and decreases their receptor sensitivity, disrupting the management of food intake and metabolism.

**Heart disease and sugar consumption.** An accumulation of scientific evidence indicates sugar consumption increases the risk heart disease. A 2002 report from the American Heart Association indicated that women who consumed diets with sweets or highly processed starches had an increase in cardiovascular disease risk. An abstract of a recent article in *The Journal of the American Medical Association* states, "Epidemiologic studies suggest that higher intake of added sugar is associated with cardiovascular disease risk factors." A study from the University of Texas Health Science Center also found that consuming too much sugar can greatly increase the risk of heart failure and explains how: "A single molecule, the glucose metabolite glucose 6-phosphate (G6P) causes stress to the heart that changes the muscle proteins and induces poor pump function leading to heart failure." Other findings suggest that insulin resistance causes lesions in the endothelium wall, causing inflammation and bringing cholesterol to the site, eventually creating "patches" that can be released into the bloodstream or that clot and block the arterial walls.

**Cancer and sugar consumption.** The link between cancer and sugar consumption is becoming firmly established. However, the suspected connection is not new. An early study (1983) in the journal *Medical Hypotheses* found a correlation in older women between breast cancer mortality and sugar consumption. A paper written in 2006, appearing in *The American Journal of Clinical Nutrition*, linked sugar with pancreatic cancer. The authors stated, "The consumption of added sugar, soft drinks, and sweetened fruit soups or stewed fruit was positively associated with pancreatic cancer."

A later study (2013) published in the journal *Cancer Epidemiology, Biomarkers & Prevention* found that the more sugary drinks a woman drank, the greater her chance of endometrial cancer. Women who drank the most sugary drinks (the authors were particularly interested in the sugar-sweetened sodas Coke and Pepsi), more than four servings per week, had a 78% greater risk of developing estrogen-dependent type 1 endometrial cancer than women who drank none.

More scientific papers are being published linking sugar consumption and cancer, but new evidence shows that sugar feeds cancer and tumor growth. In a paper published in the journal *Molecular Systems Biology*, the author found that depriving cancer cells of glucose leads to cancer cell deaths.

A study published in the journal *Molecular Cell* linked cancer and excess sugar consumption and noted that the diabetic population has up to double the chances of suffering from pancreatic or colon cancer, among other cancers. The authors discovered a key mechanism in the intestines that is implicated in the cancer progression. Dr. Costodia Garcia, the lead author, said, "We were surprised to realize that changes in our metabolism caused by dietary sugar impact our cancer risk." He went on to say, "Changing diet is one of the easiest prevention strategies that can potentially save a lot of suffering and money."

**Your brain on sugar.** Diabetes is a risk factor of dementia. In an article published in the journal *Neurology,* the authors stated that they found that people with diabetes were twice as likely as those without diabetes to develop Alzheimer's disease and other types of dementia, such as vascular dementia. Vascular dementia occurs when damaged blood vessels limit the amount of oxygen to the brain. People with type 2 diabetes also show brain shrinkage that resembles patterns seen in people with early stages of Alzheimer's disease. Another study found that people who lost brain cells were more likely to develop dementia.

It is not only those people with diabetes who may experience brain shrinkage. Several studies in the journal *Neurology* found that even people whose blood sugar measured on the high end of normal experienced 6 to 10% brain shrinkage. Another study suggested that lowering blood sugar to within the normal range is a promising strategy for preventing memory problems and cognitive decline as people age.

## Glycemic Index

Glycemic index is one way to monitor the impact of sugar intake on blood sugar levels. Glycemic index is a measure of how foods affect the glucose level in the blood. Each food is assigned a number. The lower the number, the more slowly the foods are digested and the more slowly glucose is released into the bloodstream. The higher the number, the more quickly the food is digested and the more quickly glucose is released into the bloodstream. As explained earlier, when blood glucose levels rise quickly, the pancreas is stimulated to release insulin to drop the blood sugar level. Constant fluctuations cause stress and interfere with energy production, fat storage, and the immune system. White bread and most breakfast cereals have a high glycemic index; most fruits, vegetables, and nuts have low glycemic indexes. Whole wheat products and some types of potatoes have glycemic indexes in the middle. Fats are not included.

Although the glycemic index may be helpful in some circumstances, it is not totally accurate for a number of reasons. Different laboratories give the same foods different weights, so the Index numbers are often based on averages. Different ways of preparing food and different varieties of plants yield different numbers. Because we don't usually eat just one food at a sitting, the glycemic load is only an approximation of a complete meal.

## Names for Sugar

Sugars come in many forms and may be hard to identify on labels. Here are some common names of sugars to look for when choosing food products:

| | | |
|---|---|---|
| Agave | Barley malt | Cane sugar |
| Cane sugar abstract | Corn syrup | Date sugar |
| Dextrose | D-tagatose | Erythritol |
| Fructose | Fruit juice | Fruit juice concentrate |
| Galactose | Glucose | High fructose corn syrup |
| Invert sugar | Lactose | Malted grain syrup |
| Maltodextrin | Maltose | Mannitol |
| Maple sugar | Molasses | Rapadura |
| Raw honey | Sorbitol | Sorghum syrup |
| Stevia | Sucanat | Turbinado sugar |
| Xylitol | | |

# How Much Sugar Is Too Much?

An average person on an average day needs about five grams of glucose circulating in his/her blood at any one time. Fruits, fruit juices, sodas, snack foods, breakfast cereals, and even food we have come to believe is really healthy contain much more sugar than we should be eating to maintain our brain health. Fresh fruit contains sugar but is loaded with fiber that slows digestion. Fruit juices also contain high levels of sugar but without the fiber, so juices go directly to glucose. Sodas have no food value and the benefits of the other products need to be considered along with their sugar content. How much sugar do you want to eat per day? Consider the following sugar content of these foods:

## Sugar Content of Common Foods

| Fruit | Portion | Grams of Sugar |
|---|---|---|
| Red seedless grapes | 1 serving | 20 |
| Navel orange | 1 medium | 23 |
| Apple | 1 large | 23 |
| Banana | 1 large | 17 |
| Strawberries | 1 serving | 7 |

| Fruit Juices | Portion | Grams of Sugar |
|---|---|---|
| 100% Apple juice | 8 oz. | 27 |
| 100% Orange juice | 8 oz. | 22 |
| Odwalla juice puree | 8 oz. | 38 |
| Mango Nectar | 8 oz. | 35 |
| Sunsweet Prune Juice | 8 oz. | 25 |

| Energy Drinks | Portion | Grams of Sugar |
|---|---|---|
| Kickstart | 8 oz. | 10 |
| Rockstar | 8 oz. | 31 |
| Red Bull | 8 oz. | 25 |
| Vitamin Water | 8 oz. | 13 |

| Energy Bars | Portion | Grams of Sugar |
|---|---|---|
| Pure Protein Greek Yogurt | 1 bar | 10 |
| MoJo Dark Chocolate | 1 bar | 13 |
| Balance, yogurt honey | 1 bar | 17 |
| Kellogg's Multi-Grain | 1 bar | 12 |

| Cereals | Portion | Grams of Sugar |
|---|---|---|
| Kashi Heart to Heart Blueberry | 1 cup | 12 |
| Nature's Path Red Berry, organic | 1 cup | 13 |
| Post Raisin Bran | 1 cup | 19 |
| Kellogg's Fruit Loops | 1 cup | 12 |
| Lucky Charms | 1 cup | 14 |

| Snacks | Portion | Grams of Sugar |
|---|---|---|
| Franz Apple Pie | 1 pie | 41 |
| Fruit Roll-Ups | 1 piece | 7 |
| Twinkies | 1 cake | 37 |
| Donettes, powdered sugar | 6 donuts | 23 |
| Snack Pack Pudding | 1 cup | 13 |

| Yogurt | Portion | Grams of Sugar |
|---|---|---|
| Dannon Fruit at Bottom, blueberry | 6 oz. | 24 |
| Brown Cow, blueberry | 6 oz. | 25 |
| Cultured Coconut Milk | 6 oz. | 25 |
| Yoplait Lite, blueberry | 6 oz. | 10 |
| Snack Pack Pudding | 1 cup | 13 |

# Artificial Sweeteners

Artificial sweeteners or nonnutritive sweeteners are products made from sugar, sugar alcohols, and chemicals. They are many times sweeter than sucrose (table sugar) and usually contain either a very small number of calories or none. They also reduce the glycemic response, decrease dental cavities, and are cheaper to produce than sugar or other nutritive sweeteners. A major benefit of artificial sweeteners is their cost of production. They are also used in weight loss because they satisfy our desire for sweets without adding calories to our diets. However, they do not provide the satiety that real sugar does. Some studies indicate they can cause weight gain and fat storage because they stimulate leptin and insulin production, two of the hormones involved with satiety and metabolism. Although the Federal Drug Administration has approved the use of artificial sweeteners, they remain controversial.

In the United States, sweeteners fall under the category of the Generally Recognized as Safe list of food additives under the 1958 Food Additives Amendment to the Federal Food, Drug, and Cosmetic Act. According to the FDA, "If a product is generally known by qualified experts, and there is a consensus among qualified experts that the product is safe being used under the conditions for which it was intended, then it is considered safe." Artificial sweeteners were included in 3,920 products between 2000 and 2005. In 2004, 1,649 new products containing artificial sweeteners appeared on the market. According to a recent report, sucralose alone is now found in over 4,500 cooked or baked products.

The FDA and the American Dietetic Association have approved five artificial sweeteners as safe food additives: saccharin, aspartame, sucralose, acesulfame K, and neotame.

**Saccharin.** Saccharin has been around longer than any of the other nonnutritive sweeteners and is the best researched. It is on the market as Sugar Twin, Sweet'N Low, and Necta Sweet. Saccharin is used in tabletop sweeteners, baked goods, jams, chewing gum, canned fruit, candy, dessert toppings, and salad dressings. In 1977 it was determined that saccharin caused bladder cancer in rats, but Congress allowed it to remain on the market with a warning that it could "be hazardous to your health." Subsequent studies have shown it doesn't have that effect on humans. People who are allergic to sulfa drugs have had an allergic reaction to saccharin products. Its primary ingredient is benzoic sulfimide.

**Aspartame.** Aspartame has been approved in over 100 countries as a general-use sweetener. It is marketed under the names NutraSweet and Equal. Aspartame is the most popular artificial sweetener on the market and is used in carbonated beverages, tabletop sweeteners, cold breakfast cereals, chewing gum, gelatins, and puddings. It is considered safe with a daily intake not to exceed 40 milligrams/kilograms/day, except for people with phenylketonuria (PKU). However, a book by H. J. Roberts, MD, *Aspartame Disease: An Ignored Epidemic*, indicates that 80% of the complaints to the FDA were about the health problems associated with aspartame ingestion. The complaints included headaches, mood disorders, neurological disorders, memory loss, irritable bowel syndrome, and others. Aspartame is made from phenylalanine, aspartic acid, and methanol.

**Neotame.** Neotame is a new version or a chemically related version of aspartame without the phenylalanine dangers for people with PKU. The FDA approved it in 2003 and it has been approved for use in Australia and New Zealand as well. It is also one of two nonnutritive sweeteners that have been approved by the consumer advocacy group Center for Science in the Public Interest. It is one of the sweetest of the entire nonnutritive sweetener products, with a potency of approximately 7,000 to 13,000 times sweeter than table sugar; so small amounts go a long way. Although it is not widely used, it appears in some soft drinks and diet foods. The same concerns hold for neotame as for aspartame. However, to reduce the risk to people with PKU, 3-dimethylbutyl is added, a dubious benefit since 3-dimethylbutyl is on the EPA's most hazardous chemical list.

**Sucralose.** Sucralose, the major ingredient in Splenda, is advertised as made from sugar. Sucralose is, in fact, derived from sugar through chemical processing. Dextrose and maltodextrin are added to increase its bulk. Sucralose has been approved as a general-purpose sweetener. Because it can be used for cooking in the same measure as sugar, i.e., cup for cup, it is highly popular. It is approved "safe" by the consumer advocacy group Center for Science in the Public Interest. In spite of its popularity, some studies have shown that sucralose affects the bacteria in the gut, interferes with the absorption of prescriptions, shrinks the thymus gland, and causes stomach cramps and diarrhea. Sucralose, according to J. Mercola, MD, author of *Sweet Deception: Why Splenda, NutraSweet, and the FDA May Be Hazardous to Your Health*, is made when sugar is treated with trityl chloride, acetic anhydride, hydrogen chlorine, thionyl chloride, and methanol in the presence of dimethylformamide, 4-methylmorpholine, toluene, methyl isobutyl ketone, acetic acid, benzyltriethlyammonium chloride, and sodium methoxide.

**Acesulfame K.** Acesulfame K has been an approved sweetener since 1988 and is the least researched of the nonnutritive sweeteners. The FDA reports it is backed by more than 90 studies. Acesulfame K is stable under heat, so it used in baking or in products that require a long shelf life, and is often blended with other sweeteners to mask its aftertaste. It is listed as an ingredient on the food label as acesulfame K, acesulfame potassium, Ace-K, or Sunett. It is used in carbonated drinks, protein shakes, and pharmaceutical products, especially chewable and liquid medications. Acesulfame K contains the carcinogen methylene chloride. Long-term exposure to methylene chloride can cause headaches, depression, nausea, mental confusion, mood problems, impairment of the liver and kidneys, visual disturbances, and cancer in humans. There is strong opposition to the use of the sweetener without further testing, but to date, the FDA has not required more tests.

**Blending artificial sweeteners.** Many products now contain a blend of artificial sweeteners to improve taste, cost, and flexibility. For example, to alleviate the bitter aftertaste of saccharin, other sweeteners may be added to mask the bitterness. Because no research has been done, nor is it required, it is unclear how the combinations of chemicals from the various sweeteners are metabolized together by our bodies.

# Other Sugar Substitutes

**Stevia.** Indigenous people have used stevia, a sweetener derived from a plant leaf native to South American, for hundreds of years. It is also used as a medicine for lowering uric acid, preventing pregnancy, decreasing blood pressure, and increasing the strength of heart muscles. Stevia is marketed under the brand names Estevia, Truvia, and PureVia, in which the sweet ingredient rebaudioside A has been chemically processed, although Stevia itself has no artificial ingredients. Bulking agents have been incorporated so it can be sold in packets or used as a tabletop sweetener or for cooking. Stevia is also available in concentrated liquid form, which is less processed. It was originally approved by the FDA as a "dietary supplement" because of the rebaudioside A, one of the chemicals that makes it sweet. There were concerns that stevia lowered blood pressure and had adverse effects on fertility and reproductive development. In 2008 it was given GRAS status, allowing it to become a food additive. It is available as a sweetener in 13 other countries, including Japan, Russia, and Brazil.

**Agave.** Agave is a sweetener derived from the agave plant that grows primarily in Mexico but also in some parts of the hot, arid United States. Although marketed as a natural product and recognized as food by the FDA, it is highly process through the use of caustic acids, clarifiers, and filtration chemicals to remove the agave nectar from the plant root. Depending on the particular manufacturer, it may contain more fructose than high fructose corn syrup, from 55 to 97%. Organic agave may have a lower fructose content, be free of pesticides, and be processed at a lower temperature, preserving natural enzymes.

Stevia and agave, in limited amounts, are considered beneficial sweeteners for diabetes, because they do not substantially increase blood sugar levels.

**Xylitol, lactitol, sorbitol, mannitol, erythritol, and maltitol.** These sugar substitutes come from berries, fruits, vegetables, and mushrooms. Their sweetness comes from the sugar alcohols contained in the foods and are extracted by a catalytic hydrogenation process. It is not commercially viable to extract the sugars naturally. These sugar substitutes are recognized as food additives and considered GRAS by the FDA. Xylitol, lactitol, sorbitol, mannitol, erythritol, and maltitol can cause cramping, flatulence, and diarrhea in some individuals.

**Natural sweeteners.** Two commonly available natural sweeteners are honey and maple syrup. Most commercially available honey has been pasteurized. Raw honey, honey that has not been heated over 117 degrees, contains enzymes that digest carbohydrates. Bee pollen, an ingredient in raw honey, has been used for thousands of years to treat a variety of ailments and to promote strength and endurance. Honey in moderation does not upset blood sugar in the same way refined sugar does. However, it should not be given to infants, as they cannot digest the bacterial spores.

Maple syrup available for the mass market has been processed using formaldehyde. Maple syrup right from the tree is rich in trace minerals and can be used for cooking and baking as an alternative to refined sugar. Health claims for maple syrup include promoting heart health, boosting the immune system, lowering the risk of prostate cancer, and others.

## Moderation or Regulation

As a nation, we over-consume sugar. As research continues, sugar's role in major diseases is moving more into public awareness. Robert Lustig and colleagues from the University of San Francisco wrote a "Comment" published in *Nature* that proposes sugar is a central risk factor in noncommunicable diseases, similar to tobacco and alcohol, and should be regulated as those substances are. Alcohol and tobacco are taxed as a means to limit their consumption, and Lustig and colleagues proposed that the same be done with processed foods that contain added sugars, including sugar-sweetened beverages and sugared cereals. They also suggest that the USDA remove sugar from the GRAS list, which allows food manufacturers to add unlimited sugar to any food. Such proposals have appeal but would be difficult to implement. Denmark proposed a tax on some sugary items, but scrapped the idea before it became law because of the problems of enforcement it presented. Sugar regulation may be an idea, like tobacco and alcohol regulation before, whose time has not yet come.

There is no doubt that sugar dysregulation causes a myriad of life threatening disorders and diseases, not only in the US, but in counties around that world that have adopted our Western diet. We are genetically programmed to crave sugar, and it's hard to resist, particularly with all the delicious sugary products on the market. However, sugar products, foods with added sugar and artificial sweeteners, if not regulated, should come with a warning label: "Beware: may be harmful to your health."

# CHAPTER 11

# Water and Salt: Essential for Life

## Introduction

THE PRIMARY ELEMENTS FOR THE SURVIVAL OF THE HUMAN body in order of importance are oxygen, water, salt, and potassium. We need oxygen to breathe. Water, salt, and potassium together regulate the water content of the body. Water flows in and out of the cells to cleanse and remove the toxic waste of cell metabolism. Potassium maintains the water pressure with the cells. Salt regulates the water content of the entire body and balances the amount of water held both within the cells and surrounding the cells.

## Water

Water is ounce for ounce our most essential nutrient. The human body is about 70% water, depending on age and sex, and although we can go weeks without food, we can only go five to seven days without water. Although our tissues seem solid, they are composed mostly of water. Not surprisingly, blood has the highest concentration of water at 83%. The heart, a dense muscle, is 70% water. Other muscles throughout the body contain 76% water. The brain, minus the fat, is 75% water. The skin is 72% water, and bones have the least at 22% water.

## Functions of Water

Water has a myriad of functions. It is the medium by which elements are circulated throughout the body and it is the solvent that dissolves the elements. Blood, with the highest concentration of water, transports oxygen, carbon dioxide, nutrients, and waste products. Water is used to digest food and to regulate body temperature through sweat. It delivers oxygen to muscles to maintain a balance of fluids and electrolytes so they can function efficiently. Water lubricates and cushions joints and protects the spinal cord. It flushes toxins from the body and prevents constipation. Drinking adequate amounts of water keeps skin moisturized and reduces the appearance of fine lines and wrinkles.

The chemical elements of water are $H_2O$, two parts hydrogen to one part oxygen. Water is the delivery mechanism that brings oxygen to the brain. It maintains the body's electrolyte levels to allow nerves to relay messages to and from the brain. Water is critical in maintaining a pH level of 7.4. When a solution is neither acid nor alkaline it has a neutral pH of 7, ideal for the brain.

Without adequate water, cells throughout the body will shrink. Water availability is detected by two types of brain sensors, one controlling drinking and the other controlling the excretion of urine. If more water is needed, the brain detects the cell shrinkage, and we experience the sensation of thirst. When the body contains excess water, the reverse processes occur, and we feel the urge to urinate. The kidneys regulate water balance and blood pressure, and filtrate waste from the bloodstream. Lack of water puts stress on the kidneys, resulting in a loss of electrolytes and a decrease in blood volume.

## Dehydration

Low to moderate dehydration can impair cognitive functioning, short-term memory, perceptual discrimination, arithmetic ability, visuomotor tracking, and psychomotor skills. Good hydration is associated with a reduction in urinary tract infections, fatal coronary heart disease, venous thromboembolism, and the death of brain tissue. In the elderly and the very ill, dehydration is a risk factor for delirium, which may present as dementia.

Dehydration is often confused with other conditions and can, therefore, become increasingly dangerous. Symptoms of dehydration include:

- Intense thirst
- Hunger
- Dizziness
- Swollen tongue
- Confusion
- Weakness
- Lack of energy
- Heart palpitations
- Inability to sweat
- Faintness

According to Dr. Batmanghelidj, author of *Your Body's Many Cries for Water*, dehydration also contributes to asthma, muscle cramps, dementia, Alzheimer's, depression, osteoporosis, and the symptoms of diabetes. He believes dehydration may be the origin of many illnesses, because it disrupts the body's finely tuned systems and stresses vital organs.

## How Much Water to Drink?

In 2004 the Food and Nutrition Board released new dietary reference intakes for water. It recommended that women consume 91 ounces daily and men 125 ounces: 80% from beverages and 20% from food. However, differences in metabolism, environmental conditions, such as extreme temperatures or dry air, and activity level are not factored in. Thirst may be the first sign of dehydration. One informal test for adequate hydration is the color and amount of urine. Urine should be plentiful and pale yellow.

Many liquids can add fluid to the body but may come with both good and bad consequences. Flavored bottled water, coffee and tea, sugar-sweetened beverages, and drinks containing alcohol all contain more ingredients than plain water.

## Bottled Water

The bottled water industry grossed a total of $11.8 billion in 2012, selling 9.7 billion gallons of water. Pictures of clear mountain streams and blue-white glaciers on bottled water labels convince consumers that bottled water is superior to tap water. In fact, says the Natural Resources Defense Council (NRDC) reporting on a four-year scientific study, "Bottled water sold in the United States is not necessarily cleaner or safer than most tap water. (p. 1) It is also much more expensive. According to a 2013 report in *Slate* "Business Insider," the cost of bottled water is 300 times the cost of tap water.

Tap water may come from surface water (lakes or streams), artesian wells, spring water, or ground water. Bottled water may come from similar or identical sources. Estimates suggest that between 25% and 40% of bottled water comes from tap water. The USDA regulates bottled water as a food product and the standards are the same as those set by the US Environmental Protection Agency (EPA). In some states, however, bottled water requirements differ from those for tap water. The NRDC 1997 report found key differences between bottled and tap water. (See chart on next page.)

The FDA does not require bottled water producers to disclose the water source, how it has been treated, or what contaminates it contains. The water bottles are generally derived from crude oil and treated with di(2-ethylhexyl) phthalate (DEHP), a manufactured chemical that is commonly added to plastics. A 2006 *National Geographic* article reported that 1.5 million gallons of oil are used annually to create water bottles. Most Americans tested by the Centers for Disease Control and Prevention have metabolites of multiple phthalates in their urine. Phthalate exposure may come from direct use or by indirect means through leaching and general

## Some Key Differences Between EPA Tap Water and FDA Bottled

| Water Type | Dis-infection required? | Confirmed E. coli & fecal coliform banned? | Testing frequency for bacteria | Filter to remove pathogens, or have strictly protected source? | Test for cryptosporidium, giardia, viruses? | Testing frequency for most synthetic organic chemicals |
|---|---|---|---|---|---|---|
| Bottled Water | No | No | 1/week | No | No | 1/year |
| Carbonated or Seltzer Water | No | No | None | No | No | None |
| Big City Tap Water (using surface water) | Yes | Yes | Hundreds/month | Yes | Yes | 1/quarter (limited waivers available if clean source) |

environmental contamination. Exposure to high doses of certain phthalates has been shown to change hormone levels and cause birth defects in rats.

New legislation is designed to make the water healthier for its consumers. A July 2013 announcement from the NRDC indicated that the FDA had agreed to more stringently regulate bottled water safety to the NRDC's standards. Water sources are now tested for E. coli and banned if contaminated. The FDA has also agreed to regulate the level of DEHP, consistent with EPA regulations.

## Tea

More people in the world drink tea more than any other beverage besides water. There are many different kinds of teas, each with unique benefits. Teas may guard against cancer, heart disease, and diabetes, and lower cholesterol and increase mental alertness. The most common teas in the US are green tea, black tea, and herbal teas.

Green tea is made with steamed tea leaves and has been widely studied. It has a high concentration of Epigallocatechin gallate (EGCG), a form of catechin and a potent antioxidant. Green tea's antioxidants may interfere with the growth of bladder, breast, lung, stomach, pancreatic, and colorectal cancers, prevent clogging of the arteries, burn fat, counteract oxidant stress on the brain, reduce the risk of neurological disorders such as Alzheimer's and Parkinson's diseases, reduce the risk of stroke, and improve cholesterol levels.

Black tea, made with fermented tea leaves, has the highest caffeine content. It is the foundation for flavored teas such as chai and some instant teas. Studies have shown that black tea may reduce the risk of stroke, lower the stress hormone cortisol, help reduce belly fat, and protect the lungs from damage caused by cigarette smoke.

Herbal teas are not teas at all but a blend of herbs such as chamomile, lemon grass, licorice, milk thistle, ginger, rosehips, jasmine, ginkgo biloba, and mint. They have the lowest concentration of antioxidants but may also have health benefits. Some of the specific health benefits are: milk thistle for purifying the liver, rosehips for fighting off colds, chamomile for calmness and to prevent complications from diabetes, and hibiscus for lowering blood pressure.

## Coffee

Coffee contains 300% more antioxidants than black tea and 3,333 more than an apple. A growing body of evidence shows that coffee drinkers may be protected from a range of diseases compared to non-coffee drinkers. More than 15 published studies have shown there is a benefit to drinking coffee for the prevention of type 2 diabetes. In one study, people who drank more than six or seven cups daily were 35% less likely to have type 2 diabetes. People who drank four to six cups were 28% less likely to have type 2 diabetes. Due to its ability to prevent type 2 diabetes, coffee drinking has been linked to lower risks for heart attacks and stroke. It also lowers the risks for heart rhythm disturbances that contribute to heart attacks and stroke.

Higher coffee consumption is also associated with a decreased risk of Parkinson's disease and a lower risk of dementia, including Alzheimer's disease. A 2009 study from Finland and Sweden showed that out of 1,400 people followed for about 20 years, those who reported drinking three to five cups of coffee daily were 65% less likely to develop dementia and Alzheimer's, compared with nondrinkers or occasional coffee drinkers. Decaffeinated coffee may have the same benefits as regular coffee.

A downside for some coffee drinkers is coffee causes a slight depletion of calcium, inhibits the absorption of nonheme iron, and increases the risk of acid reflux. Coffee, because of the caffeine, it is an energy booster for many people, but for others, it's a source of jitteriness. Reducing coffee intake can cause withdrawal headaches. Research mentioned in this chapter is based on self-reports of the number of cups of coffee consumed and may also reflect the lifestyle, such as better diets, more exercise, or protective genes of the coffee drinkers.

Coffee drinks can contain many calories. For example, a medium café latte (16 ounces) made with whole milk has 265 calories.

## Sugar-Sweetened Drinks

Soft drinks and sodas are sugar-sweetened drinks full of empty calories. According to *The American Journal of Clinical Nutrition*:

> Consumption of sugar sweetened drinks, particularly carbonated soft drinks, may be a key contributor to the epidemic of overweight and obesity, by virtue of these beverages' high added sugar content, low satiety, and incomplete compensation for total energy.

Many sugar-sweetened drinks also contain coloring that may be carcinogenic and other additives, such as brominated vegetable oil (BVO), that are banned in more than 100 countries. Calories for 12-ounce sodas and colas range from 140 to 160. Diet sodas contain sugar substitutes that may contribute more to obesity than the sugary drinks.

Fruit juices with their natural sweetness also contain high amounts of sugar, and without the fiber of the fruit, raise insulin levels as sodas do. Most juices are pasteurized, so they have lost many nutrients, and although labeled 100% juice, many have additives. Juices labeled "drinks" may contain very little fruit, but get their flavor and appearance from sugar, artificial flavoring, and coloring. Calories for a 12-ounce juice or fruit drink range from 170 to 190.

Energy and sport drinks have become increasingly popular and their consumption is on the rise. Although these drinks boost energy, they can have serious side effects. According to a 2013 Medical News Today report, 18 people died from energy drinks in the fall of 2012. A recent government survey indicated that from 2007 to 2011 the number of emergency department visits related to energy drink consumption increased from 10,068 to 20,783. Most of the identified patients were between the ages of 18 and 25. Energy drink consumption causes insomnia, migraine headaches, seizures, rapid heartbeat, and even heart attacks. The drinks contain high amounts of additives, such as caffeine, taurine, vitamins, and sugars. The FDA has issued a statement saying the agency will conduct a full review of energy drinks and their impact on public health in 2015.

## Alcoholic Beverages

Beer, wine, and hard liquor in moderation appear to improve memory in mice and lower the risk of Alzheimer's in people, although lifestyle may account for some results. People who drink in moderation may also moderate other areas of their lives. On the plus side, alcohol has some antioxidant qualities and may help protect the brain. The resveratrol in wine is believed to increase the lifespan in animals, although the quantity needed is prohibitive in people.

On the negative side, excessive consumption of alcohol causes difficulty walking, blurred vision, slurred speech, slowed reaction times, and impaired memory. Alcohol can produce detectable impairments in memory with only a few drinks, and as the amount of alcohol increases, so does the degree of impairment. Women's brains seem to be more sensitive to alcohol's effects than men's. Regardless of sex, excessive drinking can cause brain shrinkage and damage the liver. Recommended intake of alcoholic beverages is one glass per day for women and two glasses per day for men.

A new study in the *American Journal of Public Health* found that alcohol is a major contributor to cancer mortality and potential life lost, resulting in an estimated 18,200 to 21,300 cancer deaths, or 3.2% to 3.7% of all US cancer deaths. Fifty-six to sixty-six percent of female cancer deaths were from breast cancer. Fifty-three to seventy-one percent of men's deaths were from upper airway and esophageal cancer. The cancers resulted in potential life lost from 17.0 to 19.0 years lost per death. The authors note that daily consumption of 1.5 drinks accounted for 26% to 35% of alcohol-attributable cancer deaths.

# Salt

Salt is essential for life itself. Our scientific knowledge of the human body reveals salt has many important functions in maintaining and promoting good health. Here is why we cannot live without it.

Salt does the following, among many other functions:

- Helps maintain acid-base balance, particularly in the brain cells
- Maintains and regulates blood pressure
- Stimulates nerve impulses to fire the neurons in the brain
- Facilitates communication between the brain and muscles to create muscle contractions
- Helps balance the body's blood sugar level
- Supports the functioning of adrenal glands
- Helps clear congestion in the lungs and nasal passages
- Aids in absorption of food particles in the intestinal tract
- Is a major component of blood plasma

Although we need salt to survive, we cannot produce it on our own. We must get it from the food we eat. Salt, along with sugar and fat, gives our food the tastes we love. Fortunately, it is readily available, so available that we have been warned that a high salt diet is a major contributor to heart disease. Processed foods, particularly, contain large doses of salt. However, it's not just the quantity of salt in our food that is a problem, but the kind of salt we are consuming. This distinction is seldom made. There are basically two categories of salt: refined salt and unrefined, or natural, salt. Refined salt has had most of the minerals removed and its molecular structure is altered through the refining process. Natural, or unrefined, salt is primarily sodium and includes both major and trace minerals, elements we need for good health.

## Refined and Unrefined Salt

**Refined Salt.** Table salt, the most common salt consumed in the US, is a processed food. Most commercial refined salt comes from salt mines and is produced by creating brine, a high concentration of salt and water. Heated to 12,000 degrees Fahrenheit to dry, the heat alters its molecular structure. As a secondary process, the natural minerals are removed for other commercial markets through a process that uses chemicals like sulfuric acid or chlorine. At this point, the salt product is 97.5% sodium chloride. Chemicals, including ferrocyanide and aluminosilicate, are added to act as moisture absorbents and flow agents and to promote long shelf life. To make its appearance appealing, it is bleached white. Some processed salt has added iodine. Too much refined salt, depleted of natural minerals, can cause adrenal exhaustion, a poor functioning immune system, and thyroid dysfunction.

**Unrefined natural salt.** Natural or unrefined salt is the most desirable form of salt, because it is harvested by evaporation, drying naturally in the sun. It retains all its vital minerals. The final product includes 84% sodium chloride and 16% naturally occurring major minerals, including calcium, potassium, phosphorous, and sulfur, and the trace minerals iron, fluoride, copper, zinc, iodine, and magnesium.

Our bodies are designed to maintain an acid/alkaline balance. The amount of processed foods we consume, which are primarily acid based, throws our bodies out of balance. The minerals in natural salts help maintain a healthy acid/alkaline base. Without the minerals in salt, the kidneys become toxic or cannot function properly. Natural salt supports the functioning of the thyroid and adrenal glands and helps all cells maintain their hydration. Examples of natural salts are unrefined sea salt, grey salt, and Himalayan salt.

## Conflicting Reports

**Salt consumption.** Too much salt can be too much of a good thing. The World Health Organization recommends a dosage of less than 2,000 milligrams per day. The American Heart Association and the 2010 *Dietary Guidelines for Americans* recommend limiting intake of sodium 1,500 milligrams per day, about the amount of a teaspoon of table salt. The average intake in the United States is 3,600 milligrams per day, well above the guidelines. Excessive salt consumption has been implicated in hypertension, heart attacks, and heart failure. It has been called "America's Silent Killer."

**The dangers of too much salt.** A recent study reported at an American Heart Association meeting indicated that eating too much salt contributed to 2.3 million heart-related deaths in 2010;

40% were premature deaths. Researchers analyzed 247 surveys on sodium consumption by adults from 1990 to 2010 to determine how salt affected cardiovascular disease risk. They concluded that 15% of all deaths from heart attacks, strokes, and cardiovascular diseases were due to excess consumption of salt. Too much salt causes the body to retain water, putting an extra burden on the heart to circulate the excess volume of water in the bloodstream. The heart must work harder, putting more stress on the blood vessels, resulting in high blood pressure. High blood pressure contributes to other disorders, including strokes, heart attacks, and cardiovascular diseases. For people with congestive heart failure, cirrhosis, or kidney disease, salt may cause serious buildup of fluids, exacerbating their illness.

Another report published in the *Journal of Hypertension* projected 280,000 to 500,000 lives would be saved by a 40% reduction in sodium to 2,200 milligrams a day over 10 years.

**The conflicting evidence.** However, there is conflicting evidence about the effects of salt on cardiovascular disease. An Institute of Medicine 2013 study acknowledged the positive relationship between higher levels of sodium intake and risk of cardiovascular disease. They also concluded that lowering sodium intake to below the level recommended by the current federal guidelines of 1,500 milligrams per day for seniors and 2,300 milligrams or less per day for younger people might also increase health risks.

In 2011 a meta-analysis of seven studies involving more than 6,000 people found no strong evidence that reducing salt intake reduced the risk for heart attacks, strokes, or death. Another study from *The Journal of the American Medical Association*, from 2011, followed 3,681 middle-aged, healthy Europeans for eight years. The people were divided into three groups: low salt, moderate salt, and high salt consumption. In the low salt group, 50 people died during the course of the study. Twenty-four people from the moderate salt group died, and 10 people from the high salt group died. The risk for heart disease was 56% *higher* for the low salt group than the high salt group. Although studies have shown that some people with high blood pressure may benefit from decreasing their salt intake, most do not experience the same benefit.

**Sodium/potassium balance is the key.** Where is the disconnect? New research indicates that it's in the sodium/potassium balance, not the quantity of salt in isolation. A July 1, 2011 report in the *Archives of Internal Medicine* reported that high sodium intake, when combined with low potassium intake, was associated with an increase in cardiovascular disease and death. The authors suggested that the ratio of sodium to potassium was a more important risk than either taken separately. This is particularly important given that the US population consumes much more sodium and less potassium than is recommended.

Similar conclusions were reached by other researchers from the Centers for Disease Control and Prevention. They analyzed information from the Third National Health and Nutritional Examination Survey Linked Mortality File, selecting 12,267 participants based on dietary information to determine their consumption of sodium and potassium, as well as the sodium-potassium ratio. People were followed for a period of almost 15 years. The authors' conclusions were, after adjusting for other variables, that a higher sodium intake was related to increased mortality from all causes, and a higher intake of potassium was associated with a lower mortality risk. However, they also did *not* find a significant link between sodium intake and cardiovascular disease by itself. The authors concluded, "Public health recommendations should emphasize simultaneous reduction in sodium intake and increase in potassium intake."

**And then there's chloride.** Chloride is a component of salt and has been largely ignored or dismissed as unimportant in the debate of "to salt or not to salt." Table salt contains equal parts sodium and chloride, and scientists at the University of Glasgow have recently discovered that having too little chloride, as well as too much chloride, can have adverse effects on your health. The body regulates the level of chloride, which plays a role in balancing fluids in the body. If it is out of balance and there is too much chloride, diarrhea, kidney problems, and over-activity of the parathyroid glands can occur. If there is too little, heavy sweating, muscle weakness, and twitching may be the result.

The researchers collected data on 12,968 patients with hypertension. They followed up on them 35 years later and found that low chloride levels could lead to a higher risk of cardiovascular disease and even death in those who already had hypertension. The researchers suggested more attention be paid to chloride as part of the salt equation.

## Processed Foods

Processed foods are a huge source of refined salt. Refined salt may come under many labels, including baking soda, baking powder, monosodium glutamate (MSG), disodium phosphate, sodium citrate, or other compounds with sodium in their name. Salt, under its many names, can be found in expected and unexpected sources. Bread and bread products, crackers, tortillas, snack chips, breakfast cereals, cookies, pizza, spaghetti, ketchup, tomato juice, frozen dinners, canned soups, processed and packaged meats, processed cheese, fast food, restaurant food, and baby foods, among many other foods, contain added salt. Almost all foods processed outside of the home will contain hidden amounts of salt. Although there has been an effort by food companies to market products labeled low or reduced salt, only the label will tell you how much salt is actually contained in the product. Seldom will you find significant amounts of potassium.

In response to the latest studies on the interplay of salt and potassium, the New York City Department of Health and Mental Hygiene has described a large-scale effort to reduce sodium intake along with an increased intake of potassium. The authors of the effort, L. Silver and T. Farley, recommend potassium content be added to the Nutrition Facts on food labels to inform consumers and to optimize potassium intake, particularly given the increasing use of potassium depleted processed foods.

However, conflicting information continues to emerge. After

the release of a May 14, 2013 report by the Institute for Medicine, the American Heart Association, in an interview by *The New York Times*, reaffirmed its position on limiting salt intake.

## Balance Water, Salt, and Potassium

In light of all available information and the recommendations by various organizations and institutes, to ensure your diet includes the healthy sodium/potassium ratio, limit processed foods and eat whole, natural foods. Leafy green vegetables, such as spinach and kale, avocados, winter squash, carrots, potatoes, grapes, blackberries, oranges, grapefruit, cantaloupes, prunes, and bananas are all good sources of potassium. Use natural or unrefined salt rather than refined salt for the healthy minerals, including the potassium it contains.

A good rule from the Center for Disease Control states, "In general, people who reduce their sodium consumption, increase their potassium consumption, or do both, benefit from improved blood pressure and reduce their risk for developing other serious health problems." Along with moderate salt and potassium intake, drink adequate amounts of water or other beverages to maintain hydration.

# CHAPTER 12

# Brain Boosters: Vitamins, Minerals, and Supplements

## Vitamins and Minerals: Essential Nutrients

OVER THE DECADES, OUR FOOD HAS LOST SOME OF ITS NUTRI-tional value. The extensive use of chemical fertilizers, the depletion of soil nutrients, and the proliferation of factory farms have reduced the quality of food available at the market. Dr. Michael Murray, author of *Encyclopedia of Nutritional Supplements: The Essential Guide for Improving Your Health Naturally*, states, "It is virtually impossible to get everything we need just to provide the minimum requirements, let alone what we need for optimal nutrition." New research supports this statement. A study from Oxford University found that it would take between 3,500 and 4,000 calories per day eating our current food to meet the minimum daily requirements for vitamins and minerals. Adding supplements may be required to meet just our basic nutritional needs.

Vitamins and minerals, unlike fats, carbohydrates, and proteins, do not provide energy to the body. Instead, they help regulate the chemical reactions that convert food to energy, building strong bones and tissue, maintaining body tissue, repairing cell damage, and strengthening the immune system, among many other functions. Vitamins and minerals are considered essential, because either they cannot be synthesized or made chemically by the body, or they cannot be synthesized in the amounts that are necessary for good health. Therefore, we have to get them from the food we eat.

Vitamins and minerals are complex compounds that provide a wide variety of benefits. Many have multiple characteristics and activities and are part of intricate feedback loops balancing many bodily functions. This chapter is a summary of the vast amount of information on these nutrients and serves only as a brief primer.

Without the essential nutrients provided by the vitamins and minerals, nutrient deficiencies will affect overall health and promote inflammation and chronic and serious illness. Most nutritionists and many doctors recommend a regime of vitamins, minerals, and other supplements to insure we are getting the nutrients we need. New studies are emerging that document the benefits of vitamin supplements.

## Sample of Benefits of Vitamin Supplements

Vitamin supplementation is now used as part of a treatment protocol for a variety of diseases, including mental disorders, neurological disorders, Alzheimer's, cardiovascular diseases, and cancer.

Vascular dementia, a type of brain damage caused by diseased blood vessels, may be slowed by antioxidants. A major study involving 3,385 Japanese-American men in the Honolulu-Asian Aging Study showed that elderly men who took supplements of both vitamins C and E had an 88% reduction in the frequency of vascular dementia compared with men who did not take the supplements. The protective effect was substantially greater in men who reported long-term use of both vitamins. The study concluded that vitamin E and C supplements may protect against vascular dementia and may improve cognitive function in late life.

Another study found additional benefits. The Established Populations for Epidemiologic Studies of the Elderly, with 11,178 subjects between the ages of 67 and 105, found that seniors who supplemented with at least 100 IU per day of vitamin E were less likely to die prematurely from any causes. The mortality rate was even lower for individuals who also took vitamin C.

## How Vitamins and Minerals Differ

Vitamins and minerals differ in their composition. Vitamins are organic food substances found only in living things. They break down into chemical compounds that are either fat- or water-soluble, meaning they dissolve in either of those elements. Unlike vitamins, minerals are inorganic substances that cannot be broken but retain their essential elements. Minerals are found in the soil and water, and we ingest them from plants grown in the soil and from the animals that eat the plants.

# Fat-Soluble Vitamins

Vitamins A, D, E, and K are fat-soluble, which means they are absorbed in fat globules from the intestines during digestion. The vitamins are then circulated throughout the body in the blood. Excess fat-soluble vitamins are stored in the body tissues. The body cannot make most vitamins, with the exception of vitamin D. Vitamin D is created through the absorption of sunlight.

## Vitamin A

**Functions:** Vitamin A is a broad group of related nutrients. There are two major categories: retinoids, found in animal foods, and carotenoids, found in plant foods. Retinoids provide immune system, anti-inflammatory, genetic, and reproductive-related benefits. Carotenoids function as an antioxidant and anti-inflammatory nutrient. Vitamin A is critical for proper eye function. It promotes cell production, bone growth, tooth development, healthy skin, and hair growth. It stimulates the immune response and is essential for the formation of some hormones. It guards against night blindness, heart disease, and strokes, and protects from cold, flu, and infection of the kidneys, bladder, lungs, and mucous membranes. Vitamin A also appears to neutralize free radicals and may slow the aging process.

**Deficiencies:** Vitamin A deficiencies can result in poor growth, insomnia, fatigue, susceptibility to respiratory infections, dry hair, and dryness of the conjunctiva and cornea of the eye.

**Sources:** It is found in sweet potatoes, yams, butternut and winter squash, spinach, carrots, broccoli, kale, romaine lettuce, cantaloupes, sweet red peppers, papayas, dairy products, eggs, shrimp, beef and beef liver, cod liver oil, salmon, sardines and tuna.

## Vitamin D

**Functions:** Vitamin D is called the sunshine vitamin, because the body makes vitamin D from sunlight by converting a cholesterol-like substance in the skin to vitamin D. This vitamin promotes the absorption of calcium, magnesium, and phosphorus for development of bones and teeth, maintains the nervous system, and promotes heart health. It protects against muscle weakness and helps regulate heartbeats. It enhances immunity and is necessary for thyroid function and normal blood clotting. New standards set by government agencies advise taking 1,000 units of vitamin D—up from the previous recommendation of 300 units.

**Deficiencies:** People deficient in this vitamin may be at greater risk for osteoarthritis, osteoporosis, and breast and colon cancers.

**Sources:** It is found in sardines, herring, salmon, tuna, beef, pork, turkey, cheese, chicken, eggs, tofu, and fortified milk.

## Vitamin E

**Functions:** Vitamin E is a blanket term for eight different tocopherols, a class of organic compounds that are fat-soluble antioxidants. Vitamin E is the primary protector of the brain, which is 60% fat. It is important in the formulation of red blood cells and the blood flow to the heart. Vitamin E supports the immune system and maintains the muscle tissues of the heart and skeletal muscles. It lowers blood cholesterol and fatty acids, strengthens capillary walls, and is vital to cell health.

**Deficiencies:** Lack of vitamin E may result in damage to the nerves and red blood cells, infertility for both sexes, and neuromuscular impairment. There appears to be a link between low levels of this vitamin and increased risk for cardiac disease and bowel and breast cancers.

**Sources:** Vitamin E is found in avocados, broccoli, leafy greens, potatoes, butternut squash, sweet potatoes, mangos, pomegranates, nectarines, almonds, hazelnuts, sunflower seeds, brown rice, eggs, herring, sardines, and turkey.

## Vitamin K

**Functions:** Vitamin K has seven different forms, from K1 to K7. The natural forms, K1 and K2 are most common. K1 is found in plants and helps liver functioning and healthy blood clotting. K2 is made by the bacteria in the gut and is taken up by blood vessel walls, bones, and other tissue other than the liver. K2 is essential for the optimum functioning of Vitamin D. As a whole, this fat-soluble vitamin is necessary to promote blood clotting and bone formation and repair, and to maintain a healthy vascular system. It plays an important role in the intestines, converting glucose into glycogen for storage in the liver. It protects the inner linings of the organs and may prevent osteoporosis. It plays a role in promoting longevity. Vitamin K2, in combination with vitamin D, plays a role in preventing cardiovascular disease.

**Deficiencies:** Insufficient amounts of vitamin K can lead to problems with insulin and glucose regulation and low bone density in women.

**Sources:** Vitamin K is found in broccoli, cabbage, cauliflower, butter, cashews, egg yolks, oatmeal, blackberries, avocados, poultry, beef, lamb, and dark green leafy vegetables such as kale, spinach, and Swiss chard.

# Water-Soluble Vitamins

The vitamin B group and vitamin C are water-soluble and are stored in the body for short periods of time and then excreted through the kidneys into the urine. Water-soluble vitamins need to be ingested daily.

## Vitamin B1/Thiamine

**Functions:** This vitamin is important for learning and brain function. It enhances blood circulation, energy levels, and the muscle tone of the intestines, stomach, and heart. It helps convert carbohydrates into energy.

**Deficiencies:** Deficiencies can cause fatigue, forgetfulness, nervousness, constipation, weak and sore muscles, as well as general weakness.

**Sources:** Vitamin B1 can be found in peas, beans, egg yolks, peanuts, wheat germ, pork, fish, poultry, and brown rice.

## Vitamin B2/Riboflavin

**Functions:** Vitamin B2 enhances circulation and promotes healthy skin, hair, and nails. It aids digestion and red blood cell production and lowers cholesterol. It helps with the production of hydrochloric acid for digestion and to produce energy from carbohydrates. Vitamin B2 enhances memory and is helpful for some mental disorders. It is necessary for the metabolism of tryptophan, one of the ten essential amino acids that the body uses to synthesize proteins.

**Deficiencies:** Lack of Vitamin B2 can result in eye disorders, inflammation of the mouth and tongue, hair loss, and slowed mental processing.

**Sources:** This vitamin can be found in broccoli, carrots, potatoes, tomatoes, eggs, dairy products, legumes, nuts, fish, pork, and whole wheat products.

## Vitamin B3/Niacin

**Functions:** Vitamin B3 promotes healthy skin, improves circulation, lowers cholesterol, and assists in the metabolism of food. It enhances the functioning of the nervous system, improves memory, helps to convert fatty acids to fats used by the brain, and is helpful for some mental disorders.

**Deficiencies:** Without adequate amounts of vitamin B3, skin eruptions, insomnia, indigestion, dementia, depression, and low blood sugar can occur.

**Sources:** Sources are beef, poultry, pork, nuts, dairy, eggs, broccoli, carrots, potatoes, avocados, dates, peaches, and whole wheat products.

## Vitamin B5/Pantothenic Acid

**Functions:** This vitamin is needed by all the organs in the body and is involved in many metabolic functions. It plays a role in the production of the adrenal hormones and neurotransmitters and the formation of antibodies. Vitamin B5 helps convert food to energy, aids in digestion, and lowers stress.

**Deficiencies:** Lack of vitamin B5 can cause certain forms of anemia, fatigue, headache, and nausea. It may also impair the functioning of the adrenal glands.

**Sources:** Vitamin B5 is found in beef, fish, pork, eggs, nuts, dairy, avocados, fresh vegetables, legumes, mushrooms, dates, grapefruit, and watermelon.

## Vitamin B6/Pyridoxine

**Functions:** Vitamin B6 is critical to many bodily functions. It is important in the creation of antibodies in the immune system, in the production of hydrochloric acid for digestion, and in the formation of red blood cells. It is necessary for the absorption of fats and proteins and maintaining normal brain functioning.

**Deficiencies:** Anemia, headaches, nausea, depression, hyperirritability, learning difficulties, and impaired memory can all result from a lack of vitamin B6.

**Sources:** Chicken, fish, beef, eggs, carrots, peas, spinach, broccoli, walnuts, sunflower seeds, bananas, blackberries, and oranges are sources of this vitamin.

## Vitamin B7/Biotin

**Functions:** Biotin is necessary for cell growth, the production of fatty acids, and the metabolism of fats, carbohydrates, and amino acids. It may also be helpful in maintaining a steady blood sugar level. Biotin is often recommended as a dietary supplement for strengthening hair and nails, though scientific data supporting this outcome are weak.

**Deficiencies:** Symptoms of deficiency include thinning of hair and a red, scaly rash around the eyes, nose, and mouth. Other symptoms include depression, listlessness, hallucinations, and tingling of the arms and legs. Biotin deficiency is rare because intestinal bacteria produce biotin in excess of the body's daily requirements.

**Sources:** Biotin is found in Swiss chard and other green leafy vegetables, and raw egg yolk.

## Vitamin B9/Folate

**Functions:** Also known as folate or folic acid, this vitamin is essential for a healthy nervous system and normal brain function. It is necessary for normal fetal development. It strengthens immunity by promoting the development of white blood cells and is necessary to maintain energy levels. Folic acid supports the adrenal glands and helps slow the effects of memory decline associated with aging.

**Deficiencies:** Depression, memory loss, dizziness, nausea, confusion, irritability, digestive disorders, anemia, insomnia, and paranoia may occur when this vitamin is lacking.

**Sources:** Good sources are lamb, beef, salmon, tuna, whole grains, spinach and other green leafy vegetables, asparagus, broccoli, avocados, squash, beans, blackberries, pineapples, strawberries, and oranges.

## Vitamin B12/Cobalamins

**Functions:** As one of the most complex of all the vitamins, B12 helps in the production of red blood cells, promotes cell longevity, assists in the development of the nervous system, and maintains the myelin sheaths that cover and protect nerve endings. It assists in learning and protects against cognitive deterioration and memory loss as we age. B12 aids in the metabolism of fats and carbohydrates and is particularly important for proper digestion so the nutrients in food can be absorbed and utilized. Vitamin B12 may also help the body control inflammation by maintaining the integrity of the neuron cells.

**Deficiencies:** Chronic fatigue, depression, digestive disorders, irritability, memory loss, moodiness, neurological damage, dizziness, and bone loss may occur if this complex vitamin is deficient.

**Sources:** Beef, lamb, shell, fish and seafood, eggs, dairy products, and brewer's yeast are important sources of this vitamin. Fruits, vegetables, and nuts do not contain significant amounts of Vitamin B12.

## Vitamin C/Ascorbic Acid

**Functions:** This vitamin has several hundred important functions. It is a significant antioxidant, attacking free radicals and protecting body tissue from oxidation. It may lower blood pressure and LDL and increase levels of HDL, and it assists with the conversion of fatty acids for optimum brain functioning. Vitamin C is also necessary for the maintenance of bones, teeth and gums, ligaments, and blood vessels, and it protects against abnormal clotting. It enhances immune function and is believed to limit the intensity and duration of colds. When ingested with vitamin E, over time, it appears to maintain cognitive abilities as we age.

**Deficiencies:** The symptoms of vitamin C deficiency are increased susceptibility to infections, bleeding gums and tooth loss, and prolonged healing time. Other symptoms include joint pain, low energy, and poor digestion.

**Sources:** Common sources are berries, citrus fruits, grapefruit, cantaloupes, mangos, papayas, squash, sweet red peppers, and green vegetables, including broccoli, kale, and Brussels sprouts. Nuts and legumes do not contain significant amounts of this vitamin, nor do meats, poultry, or fish.

# Minerals

Unlike vitamins, which are organic substances, minerals are chemical elements. This means they are substances that cannot be broken down or decomposed into simpler substances by ordinary chemical processes. Elements are the fundamental materials of which all matter is composed. Think periodic table.

We ingest minerals from the plants and animal products we eat. The minerals are passed on to us by the plants, plant-eating animals, and seafood we consume. Each absorbs minerals from soil and water and passes them on to us during our digestive processes. The amount of minerals available in food depends on the soil in which plants are grown and the mineral content of the feed eaten by animals. In areas where the mineral content of the soil is low, or if our diet does not contain a sufficient variety of food, supplementation may be necessary to get the required mineral amounts for maximum health.

We need minerals to maintain proper water and chemical balance within our bodies and for the proper functioning and structure of our cells. Minerals are necessary for the proper utilization of vitamins and other nutrients we ingest. Minerals transport oxygen though the blood, regulate the nervous system, stimulate growth, produce energy, and maintain and repair bones and tissue.

Any mineral we need over 100 milligrams of is considered a macromineral. Minerals we need fewer milligrams of are called trace minerals, microminerals, or trace elements. Smaller numbers do not mean they are less important. It means we need less of them.

# Macrominerals

## Calcium

**Functions:** Calcium builds bones and teeth, helps with the functioning of muscles, heart, and nerves, aids in blood clotting, regulates the passage of nutrients in and out of cells, and reduces cramps.

**Deficiencies:** Lack of calcium can cause muscle and abdominal pain, kidney stones, high blood pressure, heart palpitations, tooth decay, cognitive impairment, and depression.

**Sources:** Rich sources of calcium are dairy foods, seafood, broccoli, green beans, and spinach.

## Chloride

**Functions:** Chloride, commonly found in table salt, is a type of electrolyte. It works with other electrolytes, such as potassium, sodium, and carbon dioxide, to keep the proper balance of body fluids and maintain the body's acid-base balance. It is an essential part of the digestive juices in the stomach.

**Deficiencies:** Deficiencies are rare but can result in headaches, tiredness, disorientation, muscle cramps, and nausea.

**Sources:** Common table salt or sea salt, seaweed, tomatoes, lettuce, celery, olives, and many other vegetables are all good sources of chloride.

## Magnesium

**Functions:** Magnesium is needed for proper brain metabolism, for building myelin sheaths for the nerves, and for controlling the balance of sodium and potassium. It converts ammonia, a byproduct of normal metabolism, into waste for elimination. Magnesium is responsible for most of the key enzymes that convert glucose to energy. It is essential for improving memory, cognitive functioning, and synaptic plasticity. Magnesium also helps maintain a healthy heart and healthy heart function by strengthening arteries. It assists in the regulation of body temperature, converts blood sugar into energy, and promotes nerve function and growth. It also promotes bone mineralization, and strengthens general immunity.

**Deficiencies:** Magnesium deficits have been linked to many brain disorders, including attention deficit disorders and age-related disorders, such as Alzheimer's disease. It may also contribute to insomnia, chronic fatigue, chronic pain, irritability, depression, cardiovascular disorders, asthma, and seizures.

**Sources:** This mineral can be found in dairy products, fish, meats, seafood, green leafy vegetables, whole grains, lima beans, bananas, apples, almonds and other nuts, pumpkin seeds, wheat germ, avocados, and spinach.

## Phosphorus

**Functions:** Phosphorus plays a role in the formation of bone and promotes tooth health, cell growth, blood clotting, heart and kidney function, and the conversion of food to energy.

**Deficiencies:** The lack of phosphorus can cause anxiety, irritability, fatigue, and low blood calcium. Deficiencies are rare, but it is important to maintain a balance between calcium, magnesium, and phosphorus.

**Sources:** The most common sources of phosphorus are meats, poultry, fish, eggs, dairy products, nuts, legumes, and dried fruits.

## Potassium

**Functions:** Potassium regulates heart rhythm, maintains fluid balance within the cells, promotes stable blood pressure, and supports a healthy nervous system. It is an electrolyte, conducting electricity in the body along with sodium, chloride, calcium, and magnesium. It is necessary to balance the effects of salt on the body. Some studies have linked low levels of potassium in the diet with high blood pressure. Others have shown that increasing potassium in the diet reduces the risk of dying from cardiovascular disease and/or stroke. There also appears to be a link between a diet rich in potassium and bone health, particularly in the elderly.

**Deficiencies:** Deficiencies of this important mineral can cause cognitive impairment, kidney failure, constipation, nervousness, insomnia, edema, glucose intolerance, muscle fatigue, and weakness.

**Sources:** Potassium has many sources, including meats, poultry, fish, wheat bran, whole grains, nuts, spinach, winter squash, potatoes, apricots, avocados, bananas, dried fruits, and figs.

## Silicon

**Functions:** Silicon is essential for the proper functioning of nerve cells and tissues, the formation of collagen for bones and connective tissue, and the growth of hair, nails, and teeth.

**Deficiencies:** Deficiencies can result in sensitivity to cold, soft, brittle nails, brittle bones, retarded growth, and thinning or loss of hair.

**Sources:** Silicon is found in whole grains, beets, rice, oats, bell peppers, and green leafy vegetables.

## Sodium

**Functions:** Sodium is necessary for maintaining the proper water balance and blood pH and for muscle, nerve, and stomach function.

**Deficiencies:** The range of problems that come from sodium deficiency include headache, heart palpations, low blood pressure, depression, dehydration, abdominal cramps, and confusion.

**Sources:** Almost all foods contain some sodium.

## Sulfur

**Functions:** Sulfur protects the protoplasm of cells against toxins and bacteria, stimulates bile function, and is important in the synthesis of collagen necessary for healthy skin.

**Deficiencies:** Lack of sulfur can contribute to premature aging, infections, and toxicity of the cells and blood.

**Sources:** Sulfur can be found in Brussels sprouts, cabbage, eggs, fish, garlic, kale, meats, and turnips.

# Microminerals/Trace Minerals

## Chromium

**Functions:** Chromium is essential for the metabolism of carbohydrates, fat, and protein. It enhances the action of insulin, helping process glucose out of the blood more quickly, promoting and maintaining normal levels of sugar in the blood.

**Deficiencies:** Symptoms of deficiency include low energy, anxiety, and fatigue due to an inability to adequately process carbohydrates, fat, and protein. Deficiencies can cause problems in blood sugar metabolism and contribute to the development of diabetes and metabolic syndrome.

Between twenty-five and fifty percent of the American population of the US population, particularly teens and older adults, is deficient in this mineral. High intake of processed food and the low levels of chromium remaining in the soil from intensive farming are the main problems.

**Sources:** Chromium is found in brewer's yeast, meats, turkey breasts, broccoli, sweet potatoes, eggs, grape and orange juice, whole grains, garlic, and red wine.

## Copper

**Functions:** Working in combination with iron, copper helps in the formation of red blood cells. It also helps maintain the health of blood vessels, nerves, bones, and the immune system.

**Deficiencies:** Deficiencies can cause anemia and osteoporosis.

**Sources:** Shellfish, organ meats, nuts, beans, dark leafy greens, dried fruits, cocoa, and black pepper are good sources of copper.

## Iodine

**Functions:** Iodine is an essential ingredient in thyroid hormones that assist with protein synthesis and enzyme and metabolic activity. Healthy thyroid function plays an essential role in brain development, metabolism, and other bodily functions. It also plays a role in our immune responses and may protect us from a variety of cancers.

**Deficiencies:** There are conflicting reports about iodine deficiencies, particularly in pregnant women. Deficiencies can cause goiter, hypothyroidism, hyperthyroidism, retardation, cognitive functioning, lack of energy, feeling cold, dry skin, among other things.

**Sources:** Iodized salt, seaweed, seafood, dairy products, eggs, and grain products are all good sources of iodine. Supplementation needs to be closely monitored, as excesses can cause toxicity.

## Iron

**Functions:** This important element is a critical ingredient of hemoglobin, the protein in red blood cells that carries oxygen to the cells. It is also a component of many enzymes and regulates cell growth. The brain cells need iron to produce myelin and neurotransmitters.

**Deficiencies:** Common iron deficiency symptoms include anemia, weakness and fatigue, slow cognitive development, difficulty maintaining body temperature, and decreased immune function. Too much iron can cause free radical damage to the fatty acids in the brain.

**Sources:** Iron is found in chicken liver, oysters and other seafood, beef, poultry fortified cereal, beans, lentils, peas, and spinach.

## Manganese

**Functions:** Manganese helps the body form connective tissue, bones, blood clotting factors, and sex hormones. It is necessary for normal brain and nerve function and to fight free radicals. It also plays a role in fat and carbohydrate metabolism, calcium absorption, and blood sugar regulation.

**Deficiencies:** Manganese deficiencies may contribute to osteoporosis, arthritis, premenstrual syndrome, diabetes, anemia, and epilepsy.

**Sources:** Common sources are whole grains, nuts and seeds, legumes, and pineapples.

## Molybdenum

**Functions:** This trace mineral is not well understood, but it is believed to be involved in many functions, including the development of the nervous system, processing waste in the kidneys, and energy production in the cells. It acts as a catalyst for enzymes and to help facilitate the breakdown of certain amino acids in the body. It may also function as an antioxidant.

**Deficiencies:** Deficiencies may cause anemia, gout, and dental cavities.

**Sources:** Common sources are beans, peas, lentils, grains, leafy green vegetables, and nuts.

## Selenium

**Functions:** Selenium is powerful detoxifier that binds with mercury, lead, arsenic, and cadmium, all of which disrupt brain chemistry by displacing important minerals such as iron, zinc, and copper. It regulates thyroid function and immune function and makes antioxidant enzymes that help prevent cellular damage from free radicals.

**Deficiencies:** The lack of this micronutrient may contribute to the development of chronic diseases such as cancer and heart disease.

**Sources:** Brazil nuts, tuna, cod, turkey, beef, sunflower seeds, eggs, whole wheat bread, rice, and cottage cheese.

## Zinc

**Functions:** Zinc is needed for the proper utilization of approximately 100 enzymes. It promotes protein synthesis, the healing of wounds, and a healthy immune function. It also regulates the activity of the oil glands and is required for collagen formation.

**Deficiencies:** Loss of taste and sense of smell, weak and peeling fingernails, acne, growth impairment, hair loss, impotence, and mental lethargy are problems caused by zinc deficiencies. It also is associated with changes in brain function and some clinical disorders.

**Sources:** Oysters, crab, beef, pork, seafood, poultry, cashews, eggs, and cheese are all good sources of zinc.

# Symptoms and Diseases Caused by Vitamin Deficiencies

Your body will often tell you if it needs more vitamins and minerals. One of the obvious signs of a vitamin deficiency is anemia, a condition that develops from the lack of red blood cells or red blood cells that don't contain adequate hemoglobin. A common symptom associated with iron deficiency is feeling unusually tired, but fatigue can also occur from insufficient vitamin B12 or folic acid.

Another telltale sign of a deficiency is changes in hair, skin, or nails. Thinning or brittle hair, cracked nails, and/or dry, irritated skin can be a sign that B vitamins and omega fatty acids are lacking. Leg cramps, particularly at night, may indicate a need for calcium, vitamin D, or Vitamin B12. Frequent minor illnesses are another sign of vitamin deficiencies. Frequent colds, flus, or general aches and pains, or minor sicknesses that linger may indicate your immune system needs support to fight off germs and viruses. Marginal deficiencies can cause minor symptoms, but if left untreated, can lead to serious problems. A blood test to check your nutritional profile can be ordered by your physician.

The connection between neurological symptoms and vitamin deficiency is emerging as a new field of study. People with Parkinson's disease, as well as schizophrenia, depression, and other mental disorders, are being treated with vitamin therapy. Peripheral neuropathy, a disorder that often occurs as a complication of diabetes, may also occur due to deficiencies of B complex vitamins, vitamin E, or omega fatty acids.

**Serious vitamin deficiency diseases.** Rickets, scurvy, pellagra, and beriberi are major diseases caused by vitamin deficiencies. Although the diseases are relatively rare, historically, they caused a variety of health problems. Today they still occur within some populations, such as those in refugee camps who do not have access to an adequate diet.

Rickets is a disorder caused by a lack of vitamin D. Vitamin D helps to control calcium and phosphate levels in the body, and when they become too low, hormones cause calcium and phosphate to be released from the bones. The result is the softening and weakening of the bones. Dental deformities may also occur. Getting sufficient levels of vitamin D and minerals will eliminate the disorder.

Scurvy is a disorder caused by the lack of vitamin C, which needs to be replenished frequently. Eating sufficient amounts of fruits and vegetables will prevent this disease. Scurvy affects the blood vessels and skin and interferes with the body's healing system. It may cause fatigue and reoccurring infections. Severe scurvy may result in vitamin deficiency anemia, leading to lethargy or fainting, uncontrolled bleeding, or rapid heartbeat. Other symptoms include spots on the skin, spongy gums, loss of teeth, and bleeding from the mucus membranes. Immediate medical attention is required or death may occur. Historically, scurvy affected sailors and others on long sea voyages where fresh fruits and vegetables were not available.

Pellagra is caused by a lack of vitamin B3 (niacin) or tryptophan (an amino acid). Symptoms are classically described as "the four Ds": diarrhea, dermatitis, dementia, and death. More specific symptoms include delusions, inflamed mucus membranes, mental confusion, and scaly skin sores. The disease occurs in parts of the world where corn or maize is a primary food source. It is also prevalent where there is little variety in food choices, such as refugee camps. Where corn is the primary food, treatment with lime, an alkali, makes the niacin nutritionally available and reduces the chances of pellagra occurring. Eating fresh fruits and vegetables will also prevent the disease.

Beriberi is a cluster of diseases caused by a vitamin B1 (thiamine) deficiency. It is one of several thiamine deficiency related conditions that may occur concurrently, including Wernicke's encephalopathy, which affects the central nervous system, Korsakoff's syndrome, which exhibits psychiatric symptoms, and Wernicke-Korsakoff syndrome, where both neurologic and psychiatric symptoms are present. Symptoms include difficulty walking, loss of sensation in hands and feet, paralysis of lower legs, vomiting, pain, and strange eye movements. In severe cases, heart failure or even death may occur. Treatment includes thiamine supplements. Today beriberi occurs most frequently in heavy drinkers or alcoholics who have poor dietary habits.

## Other Supplements

Many nutritionists and medical providers recommend other supplements in addition to vitamin and mineral supplementation. Four of the most often commonly recommended are omega-3 fatty acids, CoQ10, a general anti-inflammatory supplement, and some form of probiotics.

**Omega-3 fatty acids.** There is much evidence, both antidotal and scientific, that omega-3 fatty acids can improve brain functioning and overall health, promoting a longer, healthier lifespan. Omega-3 fatty acids are not made by the body and must be consumed in our food. The fatty acids EPA and DHA are found primarily in certain fish. The fatty acid ALA is found in plant sources like nuts and seeds. Omega-3s can also promote the genetic expression of BDNF, which contributes to the growth, integrity, and maintenance of the adult nervous system. Many diets do not contain adequate amounts of Omega 3s, so supplementation is often recommended. Omega-3 supplements are available in liquid and capsule form.

**Coenzyme Q10.** CoQ10 is a dietary supplement similar to a vitamin. In its natural form it is made by the body and found in all cells. The cells use CoQ10 to produce energy for cell growth and maintenance. It helps protect the heart and skeletal muscles and functions as an antioxidant. Studies have shown that coenzyme Q10 helps reduce heart failure symptoms and counteracts the negative effects of statin drugs. Many doctors recommend CoQ10 as a supplement when they prescribe a cholesterol-lowering drug, because the statins can reduce serum levels of CoQ10 by up to 40%. CoQ10 is naturally present in small amounts in a wide variety of foods, but levels are particularly high in organ meats, such as hearts, livers, and kidneys, as well as beef, soy oil, sardines, mackerel, and peanuts.

**Anti-inflammatory supplements.** Vitamins C and E, along with omega-3s and CoQ10, have anti-inflammatory properties. Some foods, spices, and herbs also have anti-inflammatory properties. Bioflavonoids, plant-based compounds, have been shown to have benefits. Quercetin, found in onions, garlic, and apples; procyanidins from grape seed extract; and resveratrol in red wine are examples of foods that have properties with anti-inflammatory compounds.

Ginger and turmeric are two spices that are powerful anti-inflammatories. Turmeric, which contains curcumin, has over 150 therapeutic traits, including antioxidant, anti-inflammatory, and anticancer properties. It is believed to inhibit the accumulation of beta amyloids in the brains of Alzheimer's patients. Other spices that fight inflammation are cayenne, chamomile, and cinnamon, among many others. Herbs like Boswellia, black willow bark, and licorice root are some common herbs that have medicinal properties. The bioflavonoids in plants, and the herbs and spices above, along with dozens of others, are available as supplements.

**Probiotics.** A consensus definition of the term "probiotics," based on the available information and scientific evidence, was adopted after a joint Food and Agricultural Organization of the United Nations and World Health Organization expert consultation. In October 2001 this expert consultation defined probiotics as "live micro-organisms which, when administered in adequate amounts, confer a health benefit on the host." About 400 types of probiotic bacteria exist naturally in the human gut and are believed to maintain the balance of microflora in the digestive system. As a supplement they are taken to reduce the growth of harmful bacteria and promote a healthy digestive system. The use of probiotics to improve the microflora of the gut has become widely popular, but more research is needed to fully document its efficacy.

# First: Whole, Natural Food

The best way to get the vitamins and minerals needed for a healthy brain and body is to eat whole, natural food. Although the nutritional value of much of our food supply is diminished, there are many opportunities to choose food that is nutrient dense. The proliferation of farmers' markets provides many opportunities to purchase fresh, organic fruit and vegetables. If not available, whole non-organic foods or frozen food is often a good cost effective alternative. Limiting processed and fast foods is also a way to increase the nutrient value of what we eat. Whatever the situation, vitamins and minerals are necessary for good health and nutrient value should guide food choices.

# Cultivate a Lifestyle That Promotes Brain Health

CHAPTER 13

# Exercise to Build a Better Brain

"**B**IRDBRAIN!" IS AN EXPRESSION FOR SOMEONE WHO IS FORgetful or acts foolishly. Because a bird's brain is so small, we underestimate its capacity. Don't be fooled by size. A lowly chickadee may find and hide thousands of seeds for the winter and remember exactly where each is hidden. To accomplish this herculean feat, the bird's brain expands 30% during the fall food storage season. In the spring, when it no longer needs this ability, its brain shrinks. So it is with us humans. If we use our brains, they grow. If we don't, they shrink. The key to our brain size is use and exercise.

People who exercise have bigger brains. Aerobic fitness, or any activity that uses the large muscles of the body long enough to raise the heart rate, is positively related to a larger hippocampus, the part of the brain that is responsible for thinking, and creating and storing memories. Conversely, people with Alzheimer's and other serious forms of dementia tend to have smaller than normal hippocampi.

As I've discussed, it was formerly believed we were born with a certain number of brain cells and that was it for life. Current research tells us this is not true. We now know a process called neurogenesis creates new cells. One of the mechanisms for creating new neurons is exercise. Exercise stimulates the creation of new brain cells and staves off the effects of what we call aging. It reduces memory loss and dementia, and increases physical and mental capacity. Exercise helps prolong life and keep chronic illness at bay.

## Exercise Guidelines

Our society is designed so we sit more that we move. In the 1960s close to half of all the jobs required physical activity. Today less than 20% do. Americans sit an average of 7.7 hours a day and watch television an average of four hours a day. Research indicates sitting more than three hours a day can shorten your lifespan by two years, even if you're otherwise active. We need to get moving. The Department of Health and Human Services' 1980 *National Exercise Guidelines* suggests:

- 150 minutes (2 hours and 30 minutes) of moderate aerobic activity each week, such as brisk walking or lap swimming
- Or 74 minutes (1 hour and 15 minutes) weekly of more vigorous aerobic activity, such as running
- Plus weight training at least twice a week to ensure that all muscles are healthy

Fewer than 80% of Americans meet these recommendations. Scientists at the University of Cambridge in England and others, using a meta-analysis of studies about exercise and mortality, found that, in general, a person's risk of dying prematurely from any cause plummeted by nearly 20% if she or he met these exercise guidelines, compared with someone who didn't exercise.

## Benefits of Exercise

Exercise has innumerable benefits. It improves overall health, brain health, and cognitive functioning. Exercise supports the creation of new neurons and enhances the neuron activity of the hippocampus, increasing the making and storage of memory. Exercise increases the brain's plasticity and reduces possible damage and shrinkage of the brain by controlling blood sugar level and type 2 diabetes.

Exercise controls weight and lowers the risk of heart disease, stroke, and some types of cancer. It helps improve sleep, memory, and concentration. Exercise promotes blood flow, increasing the availability of glucose, which is essential for cell life. More blood flow carries more oxygen to feed brain cells. Higher levels of fitness relate directly to positive mood and lower levels of anxiety and stress.

Even moderate exercise is better than sitting. One study followed elderly people from two to five years and compared those who didn't exercise at all to those whose lifestyles had only moderate activity. The moderate activities were household tasks such as cooking, cleaning, laundry, and gardening, and walks around the block. Those who were moderately active showed almost no decline in cognitive functioning. Those who were sedentary scored significantly worse each year. Elderly, inactive people also have fewer brain connections than those who regularly exercise. Lack of exercise accounts for 18 to 20% of preventable deaths.

But even more is going on. Our bodies are designed to move, and as we move, hormones are released. Different movements send different messages to our brains to release specific hormones, which tell the cells to burn fat or sugar, repair or build muscles, make new blood vessels, increase blood flow, increase or decrease heart rate, or increase the levels of serotonin, norepinephrine, or dopamine, which are the transmitters that provide the messages. As we exercise, we amp up these functions and move them from maintenance and survival mode to creation and building mode.

As we age, our immune systems are depressed, but exercise also boosts the immune system. Even moderate activity levels activate the immune system's T cells, which attack bacterial and viral infections. Exercise can also alter the way genes express themselves, changing how they function and interact with cells. By exercising and triggering the exercise-gene interaction, you can combat inflammation, reduce oxidation, strengthen your cardiovascular system, and slow down the aging process.

# Neurogenesis, Insulin-Like Growth Factor and BDNF

Neurogenesis, discussed in Chapter 4, is the regeneration of new brain cells, a process that it is promoted by exercise. Scientists are just beginning to understand that exercise also produces proteins that travel through the bloodstream and into the brain, playing a critical role in our highest thought processes. Insulin-like growth factor is a protein that is essential for the development and function of organs such as the brain, liver, and kidneys. It plays a role in natal neural development, including neurogenesis and dendritic branching. Moving our muscles also produces brain-derived neurotrophic factor in the hippocampus. BDNF builds and maintains the infrastructure of the brain. It plays a role in neurogenesis and the repair of synapses.

People learn 20% faster after exercise than they do before exercise, and the rate of learning correlates directly with the levels of BDNF. The production of BDNF improves overall brain functioning and may prevent or delay neurological diseases, including Alzheimer's and Parkinson's. A recent study indicated that physical exercise several times a week over a two-year period lowered a person's future risk for memory decline by 46%.

# What Kind of Exercise Works Best?

A report published in the journal *Nature Communications* described a study from the University of Pittsburgh that followed 120 seniors who were placed in two groups. One walked for 40 minutes three times a week. The other group did toning and stretching exercises. After a series of brain scans, the researchers found that the walking group experienced an increase in the size of their brains over a one-year period. The other group did not.

A second study published in the journal *Stroke* found that walking at least three hours per week reduced the stroke risk in women better than inactivity, and walking was more effective than high intensity cardiovascular exercise or moderate to heavy exercise. The same was not true for men. An article in the journal *Neurology* found that high intensity exercise in men reduced stroke risk and helped them recover from a stroke better and faster.

Nurses' Health Study data revealed that long-term physical activity, including walking, is associated with significantly better cognitive function and less cognitive decline in older women. Researchers examining data for 18,766 women between the ages of 70 and 81 found that the more active the women were the less cognitive decline they experienced. Even walking about an hour and a half a week showed modest benefits.

Long periods of sitting do more than keep us inactive. Gretchen Reynolds in her book *The First 20 Minutes* recommends standing 2 minutes for every 20 minutes of sitting. Sitting for long periods of time causes fat to accumulate in the liver, heart, and brain and contributes to weight gain and diabetes. Although the federal guidelines recommend 30 minutes of moderate exercise every day, Reynolds suggests intermittent exercise is more helpful because it changes how your body responds physiologically. She recommends walking as the ideal exercise because it's low impact and has a low risk for injury. Walking also increases circulation to the brain, and unlike more strenuous exercise, walking doesn't divert extra oxygen or glucose to the muscles.

Dr. Joan Vernikos in her book *Sitting Kills, Moving Heals: How Everyday Movement Will Prevent Pain, Illness, and Early Death— And Exercise Alone Won't* uses information from her NASA research on how weightlessness weakened the astronauts' muscles, bones, and overall health. She suggests activities that challenge gravity, such as standing up frequently if you are sedentary or must sit for long periods for your work. She found that stretching, walking, and dancing are the most effective and will produce better outcomes for maintaining fitness and health than diet and exercise plans.

Dr. John Ratey, in his book *Spark: Revolutionary New Science of Exercise and the Brain,* expresses another point of view. He states:

If you are middle age and begin exercising at moderate intensity, which means you're sweating and a little breathless for 30 or 40 minutes a day, three or four times a week, you will push back cognitive decline by 10–15 years. Some studies say the same kind of regiment can cut the incidence of Alzheimer's disease in your life by about a third.

An alternative approach to cardiovascular exercise, such as swimming, jogging, or treadmill exercise, is high intensity interval training (HIIT). It involves repeated exercise at high intensity, as hard and fast as possible, for 30 seconds to several minutes, separated by one to five minutes of recovery (either no or low intensity exercise) repeated four to six times. This form of exercise has been shown to not only decrease total cholesterol and LDL cholesterol, it increases HDL cholesterol and improves blood pressure and glucose regulation. HIIT is also effective for burning subcutaneous fat, especially abdominal fat, as well as reducing total body mass. It also improves endothelium function, those cells that form a single layer lining various organs and cavities of the body, especially the blood vessels, heart, and lymphatic vessels.

Most individuals, including those with coronary artery disease, can use HIIT safely. Some studies report a higher compliance rate with HIIT than with a standard exercise protocol, because it takes less time. However, high levels of motivation are required and the long-term benefits have not yet been thoroughly established.

A common misconception of aging is that we become increasingly frail. Exercise, depending on level of effort, makes it possible to not only maintain muscle mass but to develop new stem cells so muscles can be repaired and rebuilt. A recent study of competitive runners, cyclists, and swimmers, ranging in age from 40 to 81, found that athletes in their 70s and 80s had almost as much muscle mass as athletes in their 40s.

All these studies indicate we are not destined to the rocking chair as we get older unless we choose to keep sitting now.

# Brain Exercises

Mental exercise, as with physical exercise, improves brain function and protects against cognitive decline. Doing crossword puzzles, learning a new language, or completing a variety of complex mental tasks challenges and maintains brain capacity. Most age-related losses in memory, as with physical strength and motor skills, come from inactivity rather than disease. It's never too soon to start. People who spent time doing complex mental tasks during midlife decreased their dementia risk by as much as 48%.

Environmental enrichment also makes the neurons sprout new dendrites. The dendrite branching from learning, exercise, and social contact prompts the synapsis to form more connections. The new connections have thicker myelin sheaths, allowing them to fire signals more efficiently.

"There isn't much difference between a 25-year-old brain and a 75-year-old brain," says Dr. Monte S. Buchsbaum, director of the Neuroscience PET Laboratory at Mount Sinai School of Medicine. His findings from brain scans of more than 50 normal volunteers who ranged in age from 20 to 87 indicated that cognitive decline is not inevitable.

When 6,000 older people from another study were given mental tests throughout a 10-year period, almost 70% continued to maintain their brainpower as they aged. Certain areas of the brain, however, were more prone to damage and deterioration over time. The hippocampus, which transfers new memories to long-term storage elsewhere in the brain, and the basal ganglia, which coordinate commands to move muscles, were more vulnerable to decline. However, research indicates that mental exercise can improve these areas and positively affect memory and physical coordination.

Developing and marketing mental exercises has become commonplace, and the web in filled with programs designed to improve overall cognitive functioning, improve memory, and increase the speed with which information can be processed. Increasing the driving abilities of older people through mental exercises is an area of special emphasis.

Education in general seems to have a positive effect on maintaining cognitive functioning, particularly when it is paired with exercise. Using neuroimaging, scientists have found that higher education levels and greater physical activity in healthy elderly subjects was associated with greater regional brain volumes on MRIs. They surmised that people with higher levels of education might be less likely to be obese, thus reducing the chronic illnesses that are associated with obesity.

Better-educated people also have less risk of Alzheimer's disease. A Case Western Reserve study of 550 people found that those more mentally and physically active in middle age were three times less likely to get Alzheimer's later in life than those who were not active. Increased intellectual activity during adulthood was especially protective. Examples of the intellectual activities included reading, doing puzzles, playing a musical instrument, painting, woodworking, playing cards or board games, and performing home repairs.

## Exercise: The New Medicine

As the benefits of exercise and its role in mental and physical health becomes more apparent, it should become a first line of intervention, both for preventing and lessening the effects of chronic diseases. The benefits of exercise are well documented by scientists. It is a noninvasive treatment that puts the responsibility for people's health in their hands. If the 80% of those who are not now active embraced the exercise guidelines put forth by the federal government, healthcare costs would plummet and we would have a healthier, happier, more productive nation.

# CHAPTER 14

# Stress Reduction to Soothe Your Brain

IN 1936 THE AUTHOR OF THE GENERAL ADAPTATION SYNDROME (GAS), scientist Hans Selye, stated, "Every stress leaves an indelible scar, the organism pays for its survival after a stressful situation by becoming a little older." He believed that stress was a major cause of disease, because chronic stress caused long-term chemical changes. Today GAS is still accepted, but we have a better understanding of what happens to the brain under stress and how we can ameliorate it.

## What Is Stress?

According to the Center for Disease Control:

> Stress is a condition that is often characterized by symptoms of physical or emotional tension. It is a reaction to a situation where a person feels threatened or anxious. Stress can be positive (e.g., preparing for a wedding) or negative (e.g., dealing with a natural disaster).

Positive stress creates an increase in adrenaline, which is experienced as excitement or anticipation. Negative stress creates anxiety and worry. Stress can also create a very strong and lingering reaction that causes physical changes in the body.

Symptoms of stress include:

- Feeling sad, frustrated, or helpless
- Fear or anxiety
- Anger, tension, or irritability
- Difficulty concentrating or making decisions
- Crying
- Reduced interest in usual activities
- Wanting to be alone/isolating
- Loss of appetite
- Sleeping too much or too little
- Nightmares or bad memories
- Reoccurring thoughts of the event
- Headaches, back pains, or stomach problems
- Increased heart rate or difficulty breathing

GAS defines three stages of stress, alarm, resistance, and exhaustion. Each is regulated by the adrenal glands. The alarm stage, causing a surge of adrenaline, is the first reaction to stress, preparing us for the fight or flight response. The second stage, resistance or resolution, is the decrease in both adrenaline and stress as the situation is resolved, followed by a period of recovery and regeneration. The third stage, exhaustion, sets in when the stress and the high adrenaline continues for some time and is not resolved. The body's ability to resist is gone because your energy is depleted and you experience a sense of hopelessness and resignation.

# The Stress Hormones

The three primary hormones that respond to stress are adrenaline, cortisol, and norepinephrine.

Adrenaline, the flight or fight hormone, is primarily responsible for the immediate reactions we have when we feel threatened. It gets us ready to act by increasing heart rate, elevating blood pressure, and making energy immediately available.

Cortisol, the primary "stress hormone," is also released by the adrenal gland. It takes minutes rather than seconds for cortisol to come into play. It keeps blood pressure and blood sugar levels elevated and depresses the immune, reproduction, and digestion systems so energy is not diverted from the perceived threat. Over time, elevated levels of cortisol produce the myriad of symptoms of stress that are dangerous to health.

A third hormone, norepinephrine, acts in a similar manner to adrenaline, increasing heart rate, blood pressure, oxygen flow to the brain, blood flow to the skeletal muscles, and glucose availability.

## Effects of Stress

A strong surge of stress hormones can damage the blood vessels of the heart and brain. If the stress continues over time, the hormones cause high blood pressure, gastric ulcers, depression, high blood sugar levels, and many other health problems. Increased blood pressure in relation to stress is associated with atherosclerosis, hypertension, and cardiovascular disease. New studies indicate that chronic stress is also related to increased incidences of stroke, particularly ischemic stroke, in middle-aged men.

## Cortisol, Chronic Stress, and the Brain

Elevated, prolonged cortisol levels and chronic stress generate changes in the brain in a variety of ways. Chronic stress can damage nerve cells, particularly in the hippocampus of the brain, impairing memory and increasing the potential for dementia. Excessive cortisol in the blood may shrink the brain's dendrites, interfering with the flow of information across nerve cells and destroying cells in the hippocampus, creating memory loss and premature aging. A 2011 study found that rats whose dendrites had eroded due to stress had higher levels of anxiety than those without stress. Another study suggests that elevated levels of cortisol in adults with post-traumatic stress disorder may actually shrink the size of the hippocampus.

Stress appears to trigger the initial symptoms of dementia. An Argentine research team found that 72% of Alzheimer's patients had experienced severe stress two years before their diagnosis. The Douglas Hospital Longitudinal Study of Normal and Pathological Aging shows that increased secretion of cortisol in the older human population is significantly associated with impairment of cognitive function during aging. Cortisol causes the neurons to become over excited, firing too frequently, burning out, and dying. As excessive cortisol destroys cells, it also inhibits the growth of new cells.

Cortisol has other damaging properties. Prolonged stress alters the connections within the brain, so instead of improving learning and memory, neurons are hardwired to respond to anxiety, depression, and the symptoms of post-traumatic stress disorder. The more we experience these emotions, the more our brains strengthen these connections. Stress causes an inflammatory response in the body, and elevated levels of cortisol diminish the immune function, making it difficult to combat inflammation. Cortisol and prolonged stress increases the fat stored around the body's organs. The visceral fat secretes hormones that contribute to inflammation.

The stress response and the excess cortisol in the blood may trigger changes in the hormones serotonin and other neurotransmitters, which may be a cause of depression. Depression causes brain shrinkage, impairing learning and memory. However, when depression is treated, cognitive functioning and memory improve. There is also new evidence that prolonged stress predisposes the brain to mental illness. Usually, it is not individual traumatic events that create changes in the brain, but the cumulative effect of many stressful events.

# How to Counteract the Effects of Stress

Brain plasticity is the ability of the brain to change over time. Recent studies have shown that the brain undergoes neurogenesis, the ability to grow new neurons. A 2012 study by Alex Schlegel demonstrated that the brain stays plastic throughout the lifespan and can change in a positive way. He states, "In many cases the brain may be just as malleable as an adult as it is when you were a child or an adolescent." This plasticity is very important to counteract the effects of stress. As the brain ages, it is constantly challenged by our stressful lifestyles. The key to successful aging and keeping the brain healthy is to balance the wear and tear on our brains with activities that repair the brain.

One of the most effective ways to repair the brain and reduce stress is to make lifestyle changes: daily exercise, a balanced diet, and a good night's sleep as a backdrop for other interventions. Most exercise reduces stress if done in moderation. However, one of the most effective exercises for reducing stress is yoga. Yoga combines exercise with deep breathing. Deep breathing fills the bloodstream with energizing oxygen and switches on the body's relaxation response. A study compared GABA levels from a group of participants who practiced yoga with those in a walking group. The yoga group reported a greater boost in mood than the walking group. GABA is a neurotransmitter that is decreased in depressed people and increased in people who take drugs like Prozac.

Another study with women who were diagnosed with severe post-traumatic stress disorder demonstrated that a 10-week yoga program significantly reduced PTSD symptomatology with the same effectiveness as well-researched psychotherapeutic and psychopharmacologic approaches. The study's authors noted that "yoga may improve the functioning of traumatized individuals by helping them to tolerate physical and sensory experiences associated with fear and helplessness and to increase emotional awareness and affect tolerance."

Another way to reduce stress is to meditate. The practice of meditation has been proven to reduce the production of stress hormones, lower blood pressure, ease anxiety, and reduce feelings of panic. A study led by Dr. Herbert Benson at the Benson-Henry Institute for Mind Body Medicine of Massachusetts General Hospital showed that twenty minutes of meditation and other methods of relaxation training resulted in changes in the cellular level that countered the damaging effects of stress. The relaxation training consisted of meditation, prayer, and yoga. Another study reported by staff at the Walter Reed National Military Medical Center indicated that as little as ten minutes of meditation a day strengthened parts of the brain associated with attention, emotion regulation, stress management, and prosocial behaviors, such as a sense of empathy for others.

Dr. Benson pioneered the widespread use of relaxation to counteract stress and also recommends tai chi, qigong, repetitive prayer, progressive muscle relaxation, biofeedback, and guided imagery.

Another proponent of meditation is Dr. Kabat-Zinn. He and his colleagues opened a stress-reduction clinic for pain relief based on meditation and mindfulness at the University of Massachusetts. Some patients reported meditation reduced their pain and others reported being better able to handle the stress of living with the pain or illness.

A congressman from Ohio, Tim Ryan, was so impressed with his experience in a meditation retreat with Kabat-Zinn that he wrote a book, *A Mindful Nation*, and secured financing to teach meditation in the schools in his home district. The congressman has also hosted meditation sessions and lectures for House members and their staffs.

Mindful meditation, as adapted from *Full Catastrophe Living* by Kabat-Zinn and reported in *Time* magazine, includes these five steps.*

1. Sit with your back straight: Let your shoulders droop. Take a deep breath and close your eyes.
2. Notice your breath. Don't change your breath, but focus on the sensation of air moving in and out of your lungs.
3. As thoughts come into your mind and distract you from your breathing, acknowledge those thoughts and then return to focusing on your breathing.

---

* Most meditation practices include these elements.

4. Don't judge yourself or try to ignore distractions. Just notice that your mind is wandering and bring your attention back to your breathing.

• Start by doing this for ten minutes a day for a week. The more you meditate regularly, the easier it will be to keep your attention on your breathing.

## When All Else Fails

Stress has its place in our world, getting us up and moving when there is a perceived threat. In prehistoric times it saved our lives as we escaped from dangerous animals. Today our threats are more likely to be interpersonal relationships, commuting in heavy traffic, economic problems, and things or events we cannot run away from. Since we cannot fight or flee, we are often left with the cortisol continuing to flow through our brains and bodies. Lifestyle changes and practices such as meditation and yoga can help us to relax and change how are bodies respond to stress. If lifestyle changes and relaxation techniques do not help reduce stress, a health or mental health practitioner should be consulted for counseling or anti-anxiety medication or supplements.

# CHAPTER 15

# Sleep to Reboot Your Brain

G OOD SOUND SLEEP PROMOTES A HEALTHY BRAIN. ALTHOUGH we are unaware as we snooze, our brain is working hard, organizing and storing memories and cleaning out toxins. Without the seven or eight hours of sleep most of us need, we lose the ability to concentrate and solve problems, to perform physical tasks, and to fight off disease. Chronic loss of sleep can lead to cognitive impairment, a precursor to dementia and Alzheimer's.

## The Nature of Sleep

Scientists are still working to fully understand the nature of sleep. What is known is that our sleep and wake cycles are controlled in the brain by neurotransmitters such as serotonin and norepinephrine. A chemical called adenosine builds up in our blood during the day and causes drowsiness. This chemical gradually breaks down when we sleep. Because neurotransmitters modulate sleep, foods and medicine can change the balance of these signals and influence how well we sleep. As we age, we tend to sleep more lightly and for shorter periods of time, even though we still need seven or eight hours. About 40 million Americans suffer from chronic sleep disorders each year, and an additional 20 million experience occasional sleeping problems.

# Sleep Stages

During the night we cycle through stages of sleep: light sleep, medium sleep, deep sleep, and REM sleep. Each cycle takes on average of 90 to 120 minutes. We cycle through about five rotations during the hours we're asleep.

**Stage 1.** We begin with a light sleep that we drift in and out of and from which we can be easily awakened. Eyes move slowly back and forth as muscles relax and sometimes even twitch, a phenomena called a hypnagogic jerk.

**Stage 2.** Eye movements stop and brain waves become slower. The body temperature drops and heart rate and blood pressure slow down, giving the heart and vascular system a rest. This is where we spend about half the night.

**Stage 3.** Stage 3 is considered the deepest sleep. Extremely slow high-amplitude waves called *delta* waves begin to appear and predominate. Blood flow moves to the muscles, and tissue is repaired. Blood pressure drops and breathing slows down. Stage three is where sleep walking, talking, or eating takes place. Since this is the deepest sleep, it's also the hardest stage to be woken from. About 20% of the night is spent in deep sleep, and it mostly happens in the first half of the night. It is the most restorative, leaving us feel fresh and alert the next day.

**REM (Rapid Eye Movement).** REM sleep usually begins 70 to 90 minutes after we fall asleep. As we enter REM sleep, our breathing becomes rapid, our eyes jerk, and our limb muscles become paralyzed so we cannot act out our dreams. Although dreaming can occur during other stages, it is during REM sleep that we experience vivid, imaginative dreams. It is often called paradoxical sleep, because the body is asleep, but the brain looks similar to how it does when we are awake.

The amount of time spent in each stage of sleep varies by cycle, with more deep sleep taking place earlier in the night and more dreaming sleep in the second half of the night. By morning, we spend nearly all of our sleep time in stages 1, 2, and REM. Sleep cycles aren't an exact science and may vary from person to person or night to night, depending on circumstances and what the body may need.

# What Happens When We Sleep

Sleep has many functions. While we're asleep our brains are less responsive to sensory inputs and it can use sleep time to take care of internal business. During this quiet time neurons communicate with each other, strengthening their connections, sorting and storing information, and reinforcing memories. It's a time for the brain to consolidate new learning.

**Sleep and obesity.** Sleep has other functions as well. People on diets who sleep well lose more weight than those on diets who have sleep problems.

Poor sleep may influence the body's ability to control food intake, contributing to obesity, hypertension, and type 2 diabetes. Sleep loss causes people to eat more. It is believed that both insulin and leptin are affected by sleep loss. Sleep loss also increases the production of ghrelin, a hormone that triggers hunger.

**Glymphatic system.** Sleep changes the cellular structure of the brain. During the day, toxins and harmful proteins accumulate as a normal process of living. The lymphatic system removes cellular waste products from our bodies, but the brain is a closed system, protected by the blood brain barrier. Scientists have discovered a whole new system called the glymphatic system, which is the brain's own unique waste removal system.

During sleep, the glymphatic system becomes 10 times more active than during wakefulness, flushing debris and toxins from the brain. To facilitate the flushing, the brain cells are reduced by 60 percent to create space in-between the cells, giving the cerebrospinal fluid more space to flush out the waste material.

**Beta amyloids and sleep.** Shorter sleep duration and poorer sleep quality are linked to the Alzheimer's disease biomarker, beta amyloids. Beta amyloids are a group of amino acids that are the main component of the amyloid plaques found in the brain of Alzheimer's patients. Scientists injected mice with beta-amyloid cells and found that the beta-amyloid cells disappeared faster in the mice when they were asleep. They speculate that sleep disturbances may contribute to or accelerate Alzheimer's disease, but more research is needed.

**Repair and renew.** Sleep is a time when the body repairs and renews itself, and many of the body's cells show increased production and reduced breakdown of proteins during deep sleep. Since proteins are the building blocks needed for cell growth and for repair of damaged cells from stress and ultra violet rays, deep sleep may truly be beauty sleep, repairing not only our bodies and brains, but our skin as well.

Good sleep also improves mood and functioning. Activity in the parts of the brain that control emotions and decision-making processes is drastically reduced during deep sleep, suggesting this type of sleep may help people maintain a positive attitude and productive work behavior while they are awake. A study demonstrated that certain nerve-signaling patterns generated during the day were repeated during deep sleep. This pattern repetition may help encode memories and improve learning.

Good sleep works in tandem with the immune system. Neurons that control sleep interact closely with the immune system. Infectious diseases tend to make us feel sleepy. Cytokines, chemicals our immune systems produce while fighting infection, are powerful sleep-inducing chemicals. Sleep may help the body conserve energy and other resources the immune system needs to fight infection.

## Common Sleep Problems

The most common sleep problems are insomnia, sleep apnea, restless leg syndrome, and narcolepsy.

**Insomnia.** Insomnia, habitual sleeplessness, or the inability to sleep affect about 40% of women and 30% of men. The problem can result from stress, jet lag, diet, or many other factors. Doctors often prescribe sleeping pills for short-term insomnia. The medication may be helpful initially but stops working after several weeks of nightly use. Long-term use can actually interfere with good sleep.

**Sleep apnea.** Sleep apnea is a disorder of interrupted breathing during sleep. It usually occurs in association with excess weight or loss of muscle tone that may come with aging. In sleep apnea, the muscles relax during sleep and the windpipe collapses. Often accompanied by loud snoring, the person's effort to inhale creates suction that collapses the windpipe and blocks the airflow for 10 seconds to a minute. As the person's blood oxygen falls, the brain responds by awakening the person enough to tighten the upper airway muscles and open the windpipe. The person may snort or gasp, then resume snoring. This cycle can occur hundreds of times a night.

Sleep apnea deprives the sleeper of oxygen and can lead to morning headaches, a loss of interest in sex, or a decline in mental functioning. It is also linked to high blood pressure, irregular heartbeats, and an increased risk of heart attacks and stroke. People with sleep apnea should never take sleeping pills, which may prevent them from waking up. An estimated 18 million Americans have sleep apnea, but few have had the problem diagnosed.

**Restless legs syndrome.** Restless legs syndrome, or RLS, is a familial disorder causing unpleasant crawling, prickling, or tingling sensations in the legs and feet and an urge to move them for relief. It is characterized by constant or intermittent leg movement during the day and insomnia during the night. About 12 million Americans have RLS. The most severe cases are found in older people, although it can occur at any age. Many people who have RLS also have a disorder known as periodic limb movement disorder (PLMD), which causes repetitive jerking movements of the limbs, especially the legs. These movements occur every 20 to 40 seconds and cause repeated awakenings and severely fragmented sleep. Both RLS and PLMD can often be relieved by drugs that affect the neurotransmitter dopamine.

**Narcolepsy.** Narcolepsy is a condition characterized by an extreme tendency to fall asleep even though the person may have had a good night's sleep. The sleep attacks, over which the person has no control, may last from several seconds to 30 minutes. People who have narcolepsy may also have a condition known as cataplexy (a loss of muscle control during emotional situations), hallucinations, temporary paralysis when they awaken, or disrupted nighttime sleep. These symptoms appear to be features of REM sleep that appear during waking. About 250,000 people have this disorder, which can be treated by stimulants, antidepressants, or other drugs.

## Sleep Problems and Brain Health

Chronic sleep problems may lead to cognitive impairment and even dementia. Women who had disrupted sleep cycles were more likely to demonstrate cognitive problems and dementia than those who slept well. Too little sleep, five hours a day or less, and too much sleep, more than nine hours, both affected their average cognitive scores over time. Women with poor sleep had a 2.5 increase in inflammation compared to men who slept poorly.

Researchers have found that both men and women in their 60s and 70s who sleep nine hours or more each night have a more rapid decline in their cognitive function than those who sleep between six and eight hours. Sleeping more than nine hours may increase the risk of obesity, heart disease, and stroke. However, lack of sleep is also associated with diminishing cognitive functioning in older adults, both male and female.

Poor sleep generally appears to worsen heart disease and increase heart attacks by boosting inflammation. Inflammation is a well-known predictor of cardiovascular health. About half of people over 65 have frequent sleeping problems, such as insomnia, and deep sleep stages in many elderly people often become very short or stop completely. This may be a part of aging, or it may result from medical problems that are common in aging and from the medications and other treatments for those problems.

Loss of sleep leads to loss of brain cells. Sleep deprivation can halt new cell production. Sleep deprivation increases levels of the stress hormone cortisol, causing fewer new brain cells to be created in the hippocampus. Studies using sleep-deprived mice demonstrate that prolonged lack of sleep led to 25% of brain cells dying in the brain stem. The researchers mimicked the sleep patterns of shift workers to get their results. Shift workers have an increased risk of heart problems, digestive disturbances, and emotional and mental problems that may be related to their sleep schedules. The number and severity of workplace accidents tends to increase during the night shift.

Impaired sleep can also increase stress-related disorders, including heart disease, stomach ulcers, constipation, and mood disorders. Inadequate sleep also accelerates tumor growth. Tumors grow two to three times faster in laboratory animals that are sleep deprived.

## Sleeping Pills and Sleeping Aids

Sleep is a problem for millions Americans and sleep medications have become big business. Although their occasional use may help us though rough spots, continued use can be a problem. There are three types of sleep inducers: sleeping pills, sleep aids, and herbal sleep aids.

**Sleeping pills.** Sleeping pills are designed to help users fall asleep and stay asleep. Most pills come from a class of drugs call benzodiazepines, which target the GABA receptors in the brain. GABA is an inhibitory chemical that has a calming effect. When its effect is magnified by the benzodiazepine, it produces sleep. Common sleeping pills that contain benzodiazepine are Ambien, Lunesta, and Sonata.

Sleeping pills have potential side effects, particularly over time. They can reduce REM sleep and deep sleep and exacerbate sleep disorders, including sleep apnea. They can also produce memory disturbances, behavior changes prior to sleep, hallucinations, and sleepwalking. Sleeping pills can also be addictive and frequent users may become dependent on them for sleep.

**Sleeping aids.** Sleeping aids are over-the-counter medicines, such as Excedrin PM, Nytol, and Tylenol PM. They contain the drug diphenhydramine, which causes drowsiness. Continued use over several weeks can cause dependence.

**Herbs and natural remedies.** Many natural sleep aids have been used for centuries, yet their effectiveness, for the most part, has not been scientifically proven. As an alternative to drugs, herbal remedies do not produce the side effects found with standard medications or over-the-counter sleeping aids, and users often find them helpful in getting a good night's sleep. There are many herbs and natural remedies to aid sleep. Three common ones are valerian, chamomile, and melatonin.

For thousands of years, the herb valerian has been used as a sedative in Europe and Asia. Although it seems to help people attain better quality sleep, studies that document its effectiveness as a sleep aid are inconsistent. The quality or ingredients of product may vary and there is no standard dosage.

Chamomile is a traditional herbal remedy that has been used since ancient times to combat insomnia. It is available in the form of tea, extract, and topical ointment. It's effectiveness as a sleep aid has not been widely researched in humans, but in animal studies it has been shown to be a safe sleep aid.

Melatonin is a hormone produced by the pineal gland in the brain and is available in a synthetic form as a sleep aid. Melatonin is believed to regulate sleep and circadian rhythms and is used to address sleep disturbances such as jet lag, shift work, and delayed sleep phase disorders. It has not been proven to be effective in treating other sleep disorders.

# Our Daily Habits Affect Sleep

Food, medicine, and exercise affect the how well we sleep. Each can influence the signals sent by neurotransmitters to the brain, changing the balance of the brain chemicals and influencing our sleep. Caffeinated drinks, such as coffee, and drugs, such as diet pills and decongestants, stimulate some parts of the brain and affect how we sleep. Many antidepressants suppress REM sleep. Heavy smokers often sleep very lightly and have reduced amounts of REM sleep. They may also wake up after three or four hours of sleep due to nicotine withdrawal. Using alcohol to relax and fall asleep may help initially but reduce REM and the deeper restorative stages of sleep during the night.

Eating a heavy meal before bed may cause tossing and turning as your body works to digest the food. Individuals with acid reflux often suffer from nighttime heartburn, which can also interfere with good sleep.

Regular exercise is important to maintaining good health, but exercising before bedtime can result in a poor night's sleep. Body temperature rises during exercise and may take as long six hours to recover. Sleep generally requires your body to start cooling down, so afternoon or morning is the best time to exercise.

# Reboot Your Brain

To improve sleep, the National Sleep Foundation suggests:

- Set a schedule and go to bed at the same time and get up at the same time each day.
- Exercise 20 to 30 minutes a day, preferably 5 to 6 hours before going to bed.
- Avoid caffeine, nicotine, and alcohol.
- Relax before bed with a warm bath, reading, or other relaxing activities.
- Sleep until sunlight or use very bright lights in the morning to set your biological clock for the next day.
- Don't lie in bed awake. Do something like reading or watching television until you feel tired. The anxiety of being awake may contribute to insomnia.

- Control your room temperature so it is not too hot or too cold.
- See a doctor if your problems continue.

Good sleep, like rebooting a computer, gives the brain time to reorganize, consolidate, and refresh itself. Chronic sleep problems deny the brain its time to do housekeeping tasks and, at worst, increase inflammation and disease. Good sleep is one of the best things we can do for our brains. We need to give sleep the attention it deserves.

# CHAPTER 16

# Love and Connection: Elixirs for Life

"**L**OVE IS OUR SUPREME EMOTION THAT MAKES US COME MORE fully alive and feel most fully human. It is perhaps the most essential emotional experience for thriving and health," states Barbara Fredrickson, author of *Love 2.0: How Our Supreme Emotion Affects Everything We Feel, Think, Do, and Become.*

A global poll released on Valentine's Day 2012 indicated that most couples identify their significant other as their most important source of happiness. Almost half of all single people say they long for a partner to find happiness. Fredrickson has a broader concept, saying love is not only an ongoing experience, but also a series of encounters between people, dear friends, lovers, or strangers. If we count on romantic love with only one person, we lack imagination and opportunity to become fully human. She says, "If you expand your belief, you can experience love many times during the course of the day by being present, aware and creating those moments of loving kindness with others."

## Love and Connection

Love comes in many forms. Most of us love our families, our friends, our work, our communities, our country, our book group, our softball team, or art, theatre, and music. The list goes on. While all enrich our lives, it seems that loving and being connected to other people adds the greatest richness to our lives. Love of others is the dearest form of connection.

This is borne out by a groundbreaking study. The Harvard Grant Study followed 268 Harvard undergraduates, classes of 1938 through 1940, for 75 years, asking questions about how these men changed over time, what they learned, and what was most important to them. The simple answer was the most important thing was not money or power but love and connection. Although money and power were important, they were less important than loving, supportive relationships over the men's entire lifespans. Relationships were the strongest indicator of life satisfaction.

There were other important findings as well. If men had love in their lives as adults, they were able to overcome the effects of unhappy childhoods. Feeling connected to their work was more important than making money or traditional success. Challenges became learning experiences if connections with others were made and maintained.

Loving relationships have health benefits as well. The durability of our connections and social relationships increase the strength of our resistance to and recovery from diseases. A number of studies underscore the effect of relationship on health.

- The National Longitudinal Mortality Study reported that married people live longer, have fewer heart attacks, lower cancer rates, and get pneumonia less often than single people.
- Women in good marriages have a lower risk of cardiovascular disease than those in high-stress relationships.
- Women with ovarian cancer who had strong connections with others had a better survival rate than those who did not.
- People who were single, widowed, or divorced, who had few close friends or relatives, and those who tended not to join social or community groups died at a rate two to five times greater than people who had more extensive social ties. This

was true for both men and women, regardless of age, income, race, or ethnic background.

Connection, being in tune with others, means social bonding and attachment, sharing thoughts and experiences, and demonstrating concern and caring. In the studies, social activities were also important. Researchers found that social, physical, and intellectual activities had a beneficial effect on cognition and a protective effect against dementia. Each activity had a separate effect but converged to provide benefits to the brain. People with connections, friends, family, and spouses, and who are members of organizations tend to live longer.

Connections to others have consequences that we are only beginning to understand. Researchers have discovered a relationship between genes and social behavior. A new field, social genomics, has begun to identify the types of genes that are affected by what they are calling socio-environmental influences, how social interaction affects human gene expression.

What was known previously was relationship affects the brain at a neuron level. During social bonding, oxytocin, the "cuddle hormone," is released. The vagus nerve, connecting your heart and brain and regulated by the oxytocin, changes your facial muscles to make better eye contact and to synchronize your facial expression with the person you are interacting with, creating a positive resonance. Positive resonance increases your self-regulation and improves your physical health and an overall sense of well-being. It creates resistance to colds and flus, lowers blood pressure, and decreases the likelihood of succumbing to heart disease, stroke, diabetes, Alzheimer's, and some cancers.

# Happiness

Successful aging comes from a positive attitude, happy and meaningful activities, and doing good things for others. People who have a positive attitude and are enthusiastic, confident, active, and alert are healthier and live longer than people who are pessimistic and have a negative attitude. Happiness reduces blood pressure and inhibits the production of the hormone cortisol. On the other hand, negative emotions stimulate inflammatory compounds. Extended periods of stress and unhappiness cause changes in the immune cells and gene expression that lead to disease.

Steven Cole, a professor of medicine at UCLA who has written extensively on aging, describes two ways of being happy: creating happy activities for yourself, hedonic behavior, and helping others, or eudemonic activities. The first involves structuring your life to be filled with happy activities, creating a sense of well-being through self-fulfilling activities. The second is to help others who may be suffering or have some disadvantage. Each way of being happy affects people differently. Although each may experience happiness, those who commit themselves to their own pleasure are more prone to infectious diseases and high levels of inflammatory expression. Those who seek happiness through helping others have higher levels of antibodies and antiviral gene expression, which protects them from infectious diseases. People who volunteer and help others will generally live longer, healthier lives.

The old adage "It is better to give than to receive" has a strong element of truth to it. When you do something for another, a good deed or a nice gift, not only does that make the other person happy, it also makes you happy. That happiness, in turn, makes it more likely that you will do the same thing again. Kindness to others spreads happiness—for yourself and the receiver.

## Meaningful Activities

Love and connection often go hand in hand with meaningful activity. Meaningful activity means work that provides social engagement as well as work. The French government did a study involving half a million people and found that for each additional year of work a person performed, the risk of dementia was reduced by 3.2%. People who retired at 65 had about a 15% lower risk of dementia compared with people who retired at 60. Work provides a rich, novel experience that challenges your brain and provides protection against Alzheimer's disease. For those who do retire, volunteer work, staying socially active, and being engaged in whatever is meaningful promotes a longer, healthier life.

## Love and Connection = Happiness

All studies point to one thing. It is our interactions with people that give our lives deeper meaning, better health, and greater happiness. Whether with a partner or spouse, family, friends, or casual acquaintances, experiencing love creates physical changes that enhance our sense of well-being and general health. Being involved with others, helping others, and having meaningful activities will create happiness and prolong our lives.

# Beyond Popular Diets

CHAPTER 17

# Prevention and Cure: A Non-Inflammatory Diet

VIDENCE IS ACCUMULATING THAT DIETS LOW IN CARBOHY-drates and higher in fat and protein reduce obesity and cardiovascular risks, two factors related to brain health. For maximum brain health, it is also important to eat a balanced diet of nutrient-dense, non-inflammatory food. Inflammation is the root cause of numerous diseases, and many foods in our Western diet cause inflammation.

Foods that are non-inflammatory are naturally raised farm animals and fish, natural fats and oils, and fresh fruits and vegetables. These foods not only prevent diseases, but also have curative properties. Common inflammatory foods are processed foods, genetically modified foods, sugar, and for many people, grain and dairy products. The *Dietary Guidelines* suggest a diet of 30% fat, the *Food Plate*, 20% fat. The remaining calories are protein and carbohydrates. New research suggests a higher fat (40% or more of calories), higher protein diet with fewer carbohydrates is more effective for promoting weight maintenance/loss and cardiovascular health.

What follows are general suggestions for foods to include in a non-inflammatory diet. The information is summarized from Chapters Seven through Ten. Foods are arranged by their primary content:

223

fats, carbohydrates, and protein, although most foods contain some of each. Kinds of antioxidant foods and high fiber foods are also included to round out the non-inflammatory diet recommendations.

# Choose Healthy Fats

A mixture of fats is necessary to maintain maximum health. The exception is trans fats, which should be avoided unless they occur naturally in whole foods. Examples of good fats to include:

**Saturated fats:**
- Beef and pork
- Chicken, duck, goose, and turkey
- Butter and lard
- Whole milk and eggs
- Coconut and palm oil

**Monounsaturated fats:**
- Olive oil
- Sesame oil
- Avocados
- Almonds and other nuts and nut butters
- Sunflower and pumpkin seeds and other seeds and seed butters

**Polyunsaturated fats:**
- Fish and fish oil
- Flax seed oil
- Wheat germ
- Walnuts

# Carbohydrates for Energy

Carbohydrates are divided into two groups, simple and complex. Simple carbohydrates should be chosen carefully and eaten sparingly, because they digest quickly and may raise blood sugar. Complex carbohydrates are an excellent source of nutrients that help maintain a stable blood sugar level.

Examples of simple carbohydrates include:

- Whole foods like fruits, potatoes, and milk
- Processed foods like bread, pasta, cookies, cakes, candy, sodas, fruit juices, and many packaged breakfast cereals

Examples of complex carbohydrates include:

- Vegetables like broccoli and cauliflower
- Leafy greens like spinach, kale, and chard
- Avocados
- Asparagus
- Legumes like lentils, beans, and peas
- Whole grains

# Proteins to Build Cells

Proteins are broken down into three categories of amino acids: essential amino acids, nonessential amino acids, and conditional amino acids. The category refers to whether or not they can be made by the body. Essential amino acids cannot be made or stored, so we must eat protein to supply them. The body makes nonessential amino acids from essential amino acids or in the normal digestion of proteins. Conditional amino acids are not essential unless a person is sick.

Animal products are the most complete proteins and contain all the amino acids. Examples of complete proteins include:

- Meat
- Poultry
- Fish
- Dairy
- Eggs

Incomplete protein must be combined to insure all necessary amino acids are present to make a complete protein.

Examples of incomplete proteins include:

- Whole grains
- Legumes
- Soy
- Fruits
- Nuts and seeds

## Antioxidant Foods

Antioxidant foods break down dangerous free radicals into harmless substances or bind with the free radicals to prevent them from attacking healthy cells. Many foods contain antioxidants, but the top antioxidant foods according to the USDA are:

**Beans:**
- Small red beans
- Red kidney beans
- Pinto beans
- Black beans

**Fruits:**
- Apples
- Berries
- Plums
- Prunes
- Sweet cherries

**Vegetables:**
- Cooked artichoke hearts
- Cooked russet potatoes

# Fiber to Promote Digestion

Fiber is necessary for digestion. A general rule is to consume 25 grams of fiber per day. Foods that contain the highest levels of fiber include:

- Black beans
- Lentils, red, cooked
- Oats, rolled, dry
- Avocado
- Kidney beans, cooked
- Kale, cooked
- Raspberries
- Carrots, cooked
- Pear
- Apple with skin
- Potato, baked, with skin
- Broccoli

# Beyond Popular Diets

Many diets or food plans emphasize certain foods or reflect specific philosophies. Low-fat diets, low-carb diets, raw food diets, eating for your blood type diets, and Paleo, Mediterranean, and South Beach diets are examples. Eating for brain health moves beyond popular diets and emphasizes eating a variety of nutrient-dense, unprocessed or minimally processed foods that promote brain health and prevent or do not create an inflammation response. Particular food groups are not emphasized, and although weight loss may occur, the primary goal is to curb inflammation.

To eat for brain health, and to minimize inflammation, know where your food comes from and how it was grown or raised. Eat fresh, seasonal, locally grown and organically or naturally raised food whenever possible. Eat frozen, or as a last resort, canned food as an economical alternative. Read the labels on processed, packaged, and canned foods for calorie and nutrient content. Read the labels on whole foods and animal products to learn how they were grown or raised. Be a conscious eater and choose foods that will keep your brain healthy for life.

# A Brief Summary of a Brain Healthy Diet

**Include These Foods:**

- Multi-colored fruits and vegetables
- Naturally raised meat, fish, and poultry
- Eggs
- Olive oil, coconut oil, and butter
- Legumes
- Whole grains
- Full fat dairy
- Nuts and seeds

**Avoid These Foods:**

- Processed foods
- Dairy products if sensitive or lactose intolerant
- Factory raised animals
- Processed meat
- Grains if gluten sensitive
- Genetically modified foods (GMOs)
- Sugar and sugar substitutes
- Unfermented soy

One person's health food is another person's poison, so pay attention to how you feel when you eat certain foods. A foggy brain and low energy may indicate a diet modification is in order. Start with a balanced diet of whole, unprocessed foods. Eliminate sugar and processed foods. Chart what you have eaten and how you feel each day for two weeks. Not satisfied with the results? Eliminate grains or dairy and see how you feel. Add or subtract foods to refine your search.

Record what you eat, when, how much, and how it makes you feel. You may have to add to your notes to determine the effects of the foods you eat one day and record how they affect you the next day.

A second approach is to eliminate one food at a time if you suspect something is a problem. Omit a food from your diet for several days and see if you notice a difference. Add it back and track the results. Repeat until you have identified problem foods.

Track your foods using the chart on the next page for at least a month to find the foods that best promote your health. Need help? Consult a qualified health practitioner who can assist you to diagnose food sensitivities and allergies. See Chapter 18 for resources.

# TRACKING WHAT YOU EAT AND HOW YOU FEEL

| | What You Ate | When | Quantity | How You Feel |
|---|---|---|---|---|
| **MONDAY** | | | | |
| **TUESDAY** | | | | |
| **WEDNESDAY** | | | | |
| **THURSDAY** | | | | |
| **FRIDAY** | | | | |
| **SATURDAY** | | | | |
| **SUNDAY** | | | | |

CHAPTER 18

# Resources

## Alternative Care Practitioners

CURRENT MEDICAL PRACTICES CONTRIBUTE TO OUR NATION'S health problems. Although the system is one of the best in the world, it is symptom and disease driven, emphasizing acute care. Most doctors are not trained, nor do they have time given current reimbursement practices, to assess the underlying causes of diseases. Intervention takes precedence over prevention.

Prior to becoming ill, a large percentage of people show warning signs, such as increased waist circumference, hypertension, or pre-diabetes. However, these warning signs may not trigger a thorough, integrated intervention. Rather than look at the whole person in the context of their environment, most medical doctors are trained to address the presenting problem and prescribe medication to address the symptoms. Most medications are a godsend, and many of us couldn't live without them, but many people are looking for ways to achieve good health without medications and the side effects they bring. Alternative healthcare is filling this need. Ideally, medical doctors will work in tandem with alternative providers. Both are important to creating a network of healthcare professions to give the broadest and most complete care. Most people are familiar with the role of the traditional medical providers, the doctors and nurses who staff hospitals and clinics. Following are descriptions of alternative approaches and practitioners who provide holistic healthcare.

## Integrative Primary Care

Integrative primary care is the incorporation of primary healthcare practitioners with practitioners from various alternative traditions into a medical practice. It combines the best in primary healthcare with effective therapies that come from Chinese medicine, naturopathic medicine, biofeedback, chiropractic, massage, nutritional therapy, and other modalities of health and healing. Integrative primary care is an attempt to understand the patient's health issue at the most fundamental level, define it, and remedy it by working together in combination with the patient to provide the most effective intervention.

## Functional Medicine

Functional medicine is an evolution of traditional medicine that shifts the focus of medical practice to the whole person rather than just acute care and an isolated set of symptoms. It is a growing field of medicine that involves understanding the origins, prevention, and treatment of complex, chronic diseases. It examines the interactions in the patient's history, physiology, and lifestyle that can lead to illness. Functional medicine integrates evidence-based traditional Western medicine with alternative or integrative medicine. The focus is on prevention through nutrition and lifestyle. It uses the latest laboratory testing and other diagnostic techniques and prescribes combinations of drugs and/or botanical medicines, supplements, therapeutic diets, detoxification programs, or stress management techniques. The emphasis is on treating and preventing illness while maintaining health and a healthy diet and lifestyle.

## Osteopathic Medicine

Like all medical physicians or MDs, osteopathic physicians complete four years of medical school in addition to special training in the musculoskeletal system. Osteopathic physicians hold to the principle that a patient's history of illness and physical trauma are written into the body's structure. Treatment consists primarily of moving, stretching, and massaging a person's muscles and joints to enhance their health and well-being by assisting their bones, muscles, ligaments, and connective tissue to function together smoothly so the body may heal itself. A majority of osteopathic doctors also use many of the medical and surgical treatments employed by other medical doctors. Doctors of osteopathy practice in all specialties of medicine, ranging from emergency medicine and cardiovascular surgery to psychiatry and geriatrics.

## Naturopathic Medicine

Naturopathic medicine is a distinct primary healthcare profession, emphasizing prevention, treatment, and optimal health through the use of therapeutic methods and substances that encourage individuals' inherent self-healing processes. The practice of naturopathic medicine includes modern, traditional, scientific, and empirical methods. Naturopathic physicians act to identify and remove obstacles to healing and recovery and to facilitate and augment the inherent self-healing process. They emphasize the prevention of disease by assessing risk factors, heredity, and susceptibility to disease, and by making appropriate interventions in partnership with their patients to prevent illness. Naturopathic practice includes the following diagnostic and therapeutic modalities: clinical and laboratory diagnostic testing, nutritional medicine, botanical medicine, naturopathic physical medicine (including naturopathic manipulative therapy), public health measures, hygiene, counseling, minor surgery, homeopathy, acupuncture, prescription medication, intravenous and injection therapy, and naturopathic obstetrics (natural childbirth).

## Chiropractic Care

Chiropractic is a healthcare profession that focuses on disorders of the musculoskeletal system and the nervous system and the effects of these disorders on general health. Chiropractic care is used most often to treat neuromusculoskeletal complaints, including, but not limited to, back pain, neck pain, pain in the joints of the arms or legs, and headaches. Chiropractic physicians practice a drug-free, hands-on approach to healthcare that includes patient examination, diagnosis, and treatment. Chiropractors have broad diagnostic skills and are also trained to recommend therapeutic and rehabilitative exercises, as well as to provide nutritional, dietary, and lifestyle counseling. The most common therapeutic procedure performed by doctors of chiropractic is known as "spinal manipulation," also called "chiropractic adjustment." Manipulation, or adjustment, of the affected joint and tissues restores mobility, thereby alleviating pain and muscle tightness and allowing tissues to heal.

## Chinese Medicine

Chinese medicine is a broad range of medical practices sharing common concepts developed in China and based on 2,000 years of medical tradition. It includes various forms of herbal medicine, acupuncture, massage, exercise, and dietary therapy. The principles, theory, and healing practices of traditional Chinese medicine postulates that the human body reflects and harmonizes with the relationships that exist within natural law. Each person is an integrated whole, mind, body, and spirit, and is completely connected to nature and affected by nature. It teaches that the physical body structures form a complex, interrelated system that is powered by a life force or energy called chi or qì that circulates through channels called meridians. Meridians have branches connected to bodily organs and functions. Disease is a disharmony of the energy within the body and diagnosis in Chinese medicine identifies patterns of underlying disharmony. Treatment using acupuncture, herbs, and other modalities seeks to restore harmony. The body is a microcosm that reflects the macrocosm, and as nature has a regenerative capacity, so do all people. Traditional Chinese medicine helps patients restore and recharge this self-healing function.

# Nutritional Therapy

Nutritional therapy is a holistic approach to nutrition counseling and education based on the philosophy that nutrition is a key foundation of health. Nutritional therapy focuses on returning the body to a state of balance through a diet of properly prepared whole foods. A nutritional therapist uses a variety of assessment methods to determine a client's health status, including a review of their health history, diet, and lifestyle. Based on this information and working in collaboration with the client, the nutritional therapist provides counseling, nutritional recommendations, and suggestions for lifestyle changes that are tailored to the individual's needs. A nutritional therapist may work in concert with other healthcare practitioners, augmenting and supporting other therapies.

# Additional Books to Support Brain Health

*Brain Health for Life: Beyond Pills, Politics, and Popular Diets* has described the current state and consequences of our diets and lifestyles. It has shown how the body functions and why food, exercise, and sleep are important. It has described the benefits and problems of certain foods. Chapter 17 has suggested a simple approach to changing your diet to eliminate inflammatory foods and create a healthier brain. The following books provide additional guidance for identifying and addressing food related problems that may affect your brain and overall health.

- Campbell-McBride, N. (2004). *Gut and Psychology Syndrome: Natural Treatment for Autism, Dyspraxia, A.D.D., Dyslexia, A.D.H.D., Depression, Schizophrenia.* Soham, Cambridge: Medinform Publishing.

- Challem, J. (2010). *The Inflammation Syndrome: Your Nutrition Plan for Great Health, Weight Loss, and Pain-Free Living.* Hoboken, NJ: John Wiley & Sons, Inc.

- Holford, P. (2007). *New Optimum Nutrition for the Brain.* United Kingdom: Piatkus Books Ltd.

- Hyman, M. (2009). *The UltraMind Solution: Fix Your Broken Brain by Healing Your Body First.* New York, NY: Schribner.

- Junger, A. (2013). *Clean Gut: The Breakthrough Plan for Eliminating the Root Cause of Disease and Revolutionizing Your Health.* New York, NY: HarperCollinsPublishers.

- Kharrazian, D. (2013). *Why Isn't My Brain Working?: A Revolutionary Understanding of Brain Decline and Effective Strategies to Recover Your Brain's Health.* Carlsbad, CA: Elephant Press LP.

- Logan, A. C. (2007). *The Brain Diet: The Connection between Nutrition, Mental Health, and Intelligence.* Nashville, TN: Cumberland House Publishing.

- Perlmutter, D. (2013). *Grain Brain: The Surprising Truth about Wheat, Carbs, and Sugar—Your Brain's Silent Killers.* New York, NY: Little, Brown and Company, Hachette Book Group.

# References

## Chapter I

Bittman, M. (2008, May 21). What's wrong with what we eat. TED Talks. Retrieved from http://www.youtube.com/watch?v=5YkNkscBEp0

Bovine somatotropin. (n.d.). Retrieved from Wikipedia: http://en.wikipedia.org/wiki/Bovine_somatotropin

Carlton, M., & Carlton, J. (2013). *Rich Food, Poor Food: The Ultimate Grocery Producing System (GPS)*. Malibu, CA: Primal Blueprint Publishing.

Center for Disease Control and Prevention. (n.d.). *FastStats: Exercise or Physical Activity* [Data file]. Retrieved from http://cdc.gov/nchs/faststats/exercise.html

Daniel, K. T. (2005). *The Whole Soy Story: The Dark Side of America's Favorite Food*. Washington, DC: New Trends Publishing Co.

Daviglus, M. L., Bell, C. C., Berrettini, W., et al. (2010). NIH State-of-the-Science Conference Statement on Preventing Alzheimer's Disease and Cognitive Decline. *NIH Consensus Stat-of-the-Science Statements, 27,* 1–30.

*F as in Fat: How Obesity Threatens America's Future 2013*. (2013, August). Trust for America's Health. Retrieved from http://healthyamericans.org/report/108/

Haines, M. (2012). Fertility and Mortality in the United States. Whaples, R. (Ed.). *EH.net Encyclopedia*. Retrieved from http://eh.net/encyclopedia/fertility-and-mortality-in-the-united-states/

*Healthy Eating Politics: Alternative Views on Food and Health*. (n.d.). Retrieved from http://www.healthy-eating-politics.com/usda-food-pyramid.html

*Heart Disease Facts*. (n.d.). Center for Disease Control and Prevention. Retrieved from http://cdc.gov/heartdisease/facts.htm

Heyes, J. D. (2011, June 6). American Dietetic Association attempting to monopolize nutritional advice. *Natural News*. Retrieved from http://www.naturalnews.com/032616_nutrition_American_Dietetic_Association.html#ixzz1RZ789VlU

Hoyert, D. L., & Xu., J. (2012, October 10). Deaths: Preliminary Deaths for 2011. *National Vital Statistics Reports, 61*(6). Retrieved from http://www.cdc.gov/nchs/data/nvsr/nvsr61/nvsr61_06.pdf

Kessler, D. A. (2009). *The End of Overeating: Taking Control of the Insatiable American Appetite*. New York, NY: Rodale Inc.

Lindeberg, S. (2010). *Food and Western Disease: Health and Nutrition from an Evolutionary Perspective*. Chichester, West Sussex: John Wiley & Sons Ltd.

*Meet Michael R. Taylor, J.D., Deputy Commissioner for Foods and Veterinary Medicine*. (n.d.). US Food and Drug Administration. Retrieved from http://www.fda.gov/AboutFDA/CentersOffices/OfficeofFoods/ucm196721.htm

Naci, H., & Loannidis, J. P. A. (2013, October 1). Comparative effectiveness of exercise and drug interventions on mortality outcomes: metaepidemiological study. *British Journal of Medicine*, 2013;f5577. doi:10.1136bjm.f5577

National Diabetes Information Clearing House. (2011). *National Diabetes Statistics, 2011*. Fast Facts on Diabetes [Data file]. Retrieved from http://diabetes.niddk.nih.gov/dm/pubs/statistics/dm_statistics.pdf

Nestle, M. (2007). *Food Politics: How the Food Industry Influences Nutrition and Health*. Los Angeles, CA: University of California Press.

Ornstein, R., & Sobel, D. (1987). *The Healing Brain*. New York, NY: Simon & Schuster.

*Overweight and Obesity in the U.S.* (n.d.). Food Research and Action Center. Retrieved from http://frac.org/initiatives/hunger-and-obesity/obesity-in-the-us/

*Report to the Nation Finds Continuing Decline in Cancer Death Rates Since Early 1990*. (2012). National Cancer Institute. Retrieved from http://www.cancer.gov/newscenter/newfromci/2012/ReportNationRelease2012

Rowe, J. W., & Kahn, R. L. (1991). The future of aging. *Contemporary Longterm Care, 22*, 36–44.

Schlosser, E. (2004). *Fast Food Nation*. New York, NY: Harper Perennial.

US Census Bureau. (n.d.). *Statistical Abstract of the United States, 2011*. Per capita consumption of major food commodities: 1980 to 2008 [Data file]. Retrieved from http://www.census.gov/compendia/statab/2011/tables/11s0213.pdf

USDA, Center for Nutrition and Promotion. (2011, February 2). *Executive Summary, 2005 Report of the Dietary Guidelines Advisory Committee* [Data file]. Retrieved from http://www.cnpp.usda.gov/dietaryguidelines.htm USDA Food Pyramid History. (n.d.).

United States Census Bureau. (2007). *Statistical Abstract of the United States: 2010. Table 107. Expectation of life and expected deaths by race, sex and age* [Data file]. Retrieved from http://www.census.gov/prod/2006pubs/07statab/vitstat.pdf Walsh, B. (2014, June 22). Don't Blame Fat. *Time, 183*(4).

Weber, K. (Ed.). (2009). *Food Inc.: A Participant's Guide: How Industrial Food is Making Us Sicker, Fatter and Poorer—And What You Can Do About It.* Boulder, CO: Perseus Books Group.

# Chapter 2

Adams, M. (Ed). (2013, February). US dairy industry petitions FDA to approve aspartame as hidden unlabeled additive in milk, yogurt, eggnog and cream. *Natural News*. Retrieved from http://naturalnews.com/039244_milk_aspartame_FDA_petition.html

Aris, A., & Leblanc, S. (2011, May 31). Maternal and fetal exposure to pesticides associated to genetically modified foods in Eastern Townships of Quebec, Canada. Reprod Toxical (4), 528–3. In Smith, J. M. (2013, September). *Can Genetically-Engineered Foods Explain the Exploding Gluten Sensitivity?* Institute for Responsible Technology. Retrieved from http://responsibletechnology.org/media/images/content/Exploding-Gluten-Sensitivity_.pdf?key=32174740

Benbrook, C. M., Butler, G., Latif, M. A., et al. (2012, December 9). Organic Enhances Milk Nutritional Quality by Shifting Fatty Acid Composition: A United States-Wide, 18-Month Study. *PLOS One, 2013, 8*(12);e82429. doi:10.1371/journal.pone.0082429

Carlton, M., & Carlton, J. (2013). *Rich Food, Poor Food: The Ultimate Grocery Producing System (GPS)*. Malibu, CA: Primal Blueprint Publishing.

Casassus, B. (2013, November). Study linking GM maize to rat tumors is retracted. *Nature*. doi:10.1038/nature2013.14268

*Child Obesity Facts*. (n.d.). Center for Disease Control and Prevention. Retrieved from http://www.cdc.gov/obesity/data/childhood.html

*Confirming The Link Between Fast Food And Depression*. (2013, April 3)

Medical News Today. Retrieved from http://www.medicalnewstoday.com/releases/243624.php

Davis, B., & Carpenter, C. (2009, March). Proximity of Fast-Food Restaurants to Schools and Adolescent Obesity. *American Journal of Public Health*, *99*(3), 505–510. Retrieved from http://www.ncbi.nlm.nih.gov/pmc/articles/PMC2661452/

Ellwood, P., Asher, M. I., García-Marcos, L., et al. (2013, January 14). Do fast foods cause asthma, rhinoconjunctivitis and eczema? Global findings from the International Study of Asthma and Allergies in Childhood (ISAAC) Phase Three. *Thorax*. doi:10.1136/thoraxjnl-2012-202285

Fallon, S. (2005). *Dirty Secrets of the Food Processing Industry*. The Weston A. Price Foundation. Retrieved from http://www.westonaprice.org/modern-foods/dirty-secrets-of-the-food-processing-industry

*F as in Fat: How Obesity Threatens America's Future 2012*. (2012, September). Trust for America's Health. Retrieved from http://healthyamericans.org/report/100/

*F as in Fat: How Obesity Threatens America's Future 2013*. (2013, August). Trust for America's Health. Retrieved from http://healthyamericans.org/report/108/

FDA Consumer Health Information. (2008) *Food Label Helps Consumers Make Healthier Choices* [Data file]. Downloaded from http://www.fda.gov/downloads/ForConsumers/ConsumerUpdates/UCM199361.pdf

Fleischhacker, S. E., Evenson, K. R., Rodriquez, D. A., & Ammerman, A. S. (2011, May). A systematic review of fast food access studies. *Obesity Review*, 460–71. doi:10.1111/j.1467-789X.2010.00715.x

Founder, S. J. (2012, March 3). *Un-Earthed: Is Monsanto's Glyphosate destroying the soil?* GreenMedInfo. Retrieved from http://www.greenmedinfo.com/blog/un-earthed-monsantos-glyphosate-destroying-soil

Hartke, K. (2011, November 17). *FDA Conceded Raw Milk Across State Lines OK for Personal Consumption*. The Weston A. Price Foundation. Retrieved from http://www.westonaprice.org/press/fda-concedes-raw-milk-across-state-lines-ok-for-personal-consumption

*High Fiber Cereals*. (n.d.). How Products Are Made, Volume 3. Retrieved from http://www.madehow.com/Volume-3/Cereal.html#ixzz2uNJPhJks

Johnson, L. (2013, June 13). McDonald's closing all restaurants in Bolivia as nation rejects fast food. *Natural News*. Retrieved from http://www.naturalnews.com/040752_bolivia_mcdonalds_restaurants_fast_food.html

Lawrence, F. (2010, November 23). Drop that spoon! The truth about breakfast cereals. *The Guardian*. Retrieved from http://www.theguardian.com/business/2010/nov/23/food-book-extract-felicity-lawrence

Lin, B., & Morrison, B. M. (2012, June). *Food and Nutrient Intake Data: Taking a Look at the Nutritional Quality of Foods Eaten at Home and Away From Home.* Economic USDA Economic Research Service. Retrieved from http://www.ers.usda.gov/amber-waves/2012-june/data-feature-food-and-nutrient-intake-data.aspx#.U0gfVhzqB_0

Ludwig, D. S., & Willett, W. C. (2013, September). Three Daily Servings of Reduced-Fat Milk: An Evidence-Based Recommendation? *The Journal of the American Medical Association Pediatric, 67*(9), 788–789. doi:10.1001/jamapediatrics.2013.2408

Muntel, S. (2012, May 3). Fast Food—Is it the Enemy. The IU Health Blog. Retrieved from http://iuhealth.org/blog/detail/fast-food-is-it-the-enemy-by-iu-healths-sarah-muntel-rd/#.U0qyWhzqB_0

Nader, R. (2014, June 20). The Food Safety Movement Grows Tall. *The Huffington Post*, The Blog. Retrieved from http://www.huffingtonpost.com/ralph-nader/the-food-safety-movement_b_5515885.html

Paddock, C. (2013, October 18). *Oreo cookies as addictive as cocaine—to rats.* Medical News Today. Retrieved from http://www.medicalnewstoday.com/articles/267543.php

Poti, J. M., Duffey, K. J., & Popkin, B. M. (2013, October 23). The association of fast food consumption with poor dietary outcomes and obesity among children: Is it the fast food or the remainder of the diet? *The American Journal of Clinical Nutrition, 99*(1), 162–171. doi:10.3945/ajcn.113.071928

Prayson, B., McMahon, J. T., & Prayson, R. A. (2008, December). Fast food hamburgers: What are you really eating? *Annals of Diagnostic Pathology, 12*(6), 406–9. doi:10.1016/j.anndiagpath.2008.06.002

Sacks, F. M., Lichtenstein, A., Van Horn, L., et al. (2006, January 17). Soy Protein, Isoflavones, and Cardiovascular Health. *Circulation, 113*, 1034–1044. doi:10.1161/ CIRCULATIONAHA.106.171052

Soybeans. (n.d.). The World's Healthiest Foods. The George Mateljan Foundation. Retrieved from http://www.whfoods.com/genpage.php?tname=foodspice&dbid=79

Spurlock, M. (2004). *Super Size Me* [Documentary film]. United States: The Con.

Stossel, R. (2013, May 23). Why fast food is not fit for human consumption. *Natural*

*News*. Retrieved from http://www.naturalnews.com/040736_Fast_Food_
Nation_processed_foods_human_consumption.html

*The Dangers of Raw Milk: Unpasteurized Milk Can Pose a Serious Health Risk*. (2012).
US Food and Drug Administration. Retrieved from http://www.fda.gov/Food/
ResourcesForYou/consumers/ucm079516.htm

Urbana. (2013, March 27). *What makes a food organic, and is the extra money
you'll spend worth it?* Department of Food Science & Human Nutrition,
ACES, University of Illinois. Retrieved from http://fshn.illinois.edu/news/
what-makes-food-organic-and-extra-money-youll-spend-worth-it

US Department of Health and Human Services and Food and Drug Administration, Center for Food Safety and Applied Nutrition. (n.d.). *A Food Labeling
Guide, Guidance for Industry* [Data file]. Retrieved from http://www.fda.gov/
downloads/Food/GuidanceRegulation/UCM265446.pdf

*What is a normal BMI range?* (n.d.). Ask.com, Health. Retrieved from http://www.
ask.com/question/what-is-a-normal-bmi-range?ad=semD&an=google_s&am=
broad&ap=google.com&o=11072

Young, A. (2014, April 18). McDonald's Q1 Earnings Preview: Profits
Seen Down 2.7%. Stock Market News. *International Business Times*.
Retrieved from http://www.investing.com/news/stock-market-news/
mcdonald's-q1-earnings-preview:-profits-seen-down-2.7-278357

# Chapter 3

Al-Kourainy. (2014, December 24). *The unintended consequences of the new
statin guidelines*. Retrieved from http://healthaffairs.org/blog/2013/12/24/
the-unintended-consequences-of-the-new-statin-guidelines/

Babyak, L. A., Blumenthal, J. A., Herman, S., et al. (2000, September–October).
Exercise treatment for major depression: maintenance of therapeutic benefit at
10 months. *Psychosomatic Medicine Journal*, *62*, 633–688. Retrieved from http://
www.ncbi.nlm.nih.gov/pubmed/11020092

Besser, R. (2013, December 18). *Outrage at the Increasingly High Cost of Cancer
Drugs*. Retrieved from http://abcnews.go.com/blogs/health/2013/12/18/
outrage-at-the-increasingly-high-cost-of-cancer-drugs/

Crowly, S. (2013, April 26). Doctors blast ethics of $100,000 cancer drugs.
CNNMoney. Retrieved from http://money.cnn.com/2013/04/25/news/
economy/cancer-drug-cost/

Gøtzsche, P. C. (2013). *Deadly Medicines and Organised Crime: How Big Pharma Has Corrupted Healthcare.* London, United Kingdom: Radcliffe Publishing House.

Harris, K. D. (2008, May 20). *$58 Million Merck Settlement To Change Deceptive TV Drug Advertisement.* Office of the Attorney General, State of California Department of Justice. Retrieved from http://oag.ca.gov/news/press-releases/58-million-merck-settlement-change-deceptive-tv-drug-advertisements

Hartman, T. (2013, April 30). *11 Major Drug Companies Raked in $85 Billion Last Year, and Left Many to Die Who Couldn't Buy Their Pricy Drugs.* AlterNet. Retrieved from http://www.alternet.org/11-major-drug-companies-raked-85-billion-last-year-and-left-many-die-who-couldnt-buy-their-pricey

Heimlich, C. (2011, October 24). Vitamin and nutrient deficiencies caused by medications [Blog post]. Retrieved from http://www.askdrheimlich.com/blog/vitamin-and-nutrient-deficiencies-caused-by-medications/

LaMattina, J., (2013, December 14). Marcia Angell's attacks on pharma have lost all credibility. *Forbes.* Retrieved from http://www.forbes.com/sites/johnlamattina/2012/12/14/marcia-angells-attacks-on-pharma-have-lost-all-credibility/

Mercola, J. (2013, October 16). *Pulling back the curtain on the organized crime ring that is the pharmaceutical drug cartel.* Retrieved from http://articles.mercola.com/sites/articles/archive/2013/10/16/drug-commercials-misleading.aspx

Mercola, J. (2014, January 8). *Glaxo says it will stop paying doctors to promote drugs.* Retrieved from http://articles.mercola.com/sites/articles/archive/2014/01/08/glaxosmithkline-drug-promotion.aspx

Naci, H., & Loannidis, J. P. A. (2013, October 1). Comparative effectiveness of exercise and drug interventions on mortality outcomes: metaepidemiological study. *British Journal of Medicine,* 2013;f5577. doi:10.1136bjm.f5577

Net Income for Top 11 Global Pharmaceutical Companies (in millions of dollars). (2013). Retrieved from http://usaction.org/wp-content/blogs.dir/4/wp-content/uploads/2013/04/DrugCoEarnings2013.pdf

Orseck, K. (2013, April 3). 1st Circuit Rules Against Pfizer in 3 Neurontin RICO Suits. *Law360.* Retrieved from http://www.law360.com/articles/430005/1st-circ-rules-against-pfizer-in-3-neurontin-rico-suits

Psaty, B. M., & Burke, S.P. (2006). Institute of Medicine urges reforms at FDA. *New England Journal of Medicine, 355,* 1753–1755. Reported in Peter C. Gøtzsche.

(2013). *Deadly Medicines and Organised Crime: How Big Pharma Has Corrupted Healthcare.* London, United Kingdom: Radcliffe Publishing House (p. 110).

Reinberg, S. (2012, November 11). *New Guidelines May Widen Use of Statins: Recommendations focus on patient risk factors rather than cholesterol numbers, experts say.* WebMD. Cholesterol & Triglycerides Health Center. Retrieved from http://www.webmd.com/cholesterol-management/news/20131112/heart-experts-warn-against-crash-diets?page=2

Rennie, D. (2013). Introduction. In Peter C. Gøtzsche. *Deadly Medicines and Organised Crime: How Big Pharma Has Corrupted Healthcare* (p. x). London, United Kingdom: Radcliffe Publishing House.

Rimer, J., Dwan, K., Lawlor, D. A., et al. (2012). Exercise for depression. *Cochrane Database Systematic Review, 7,* CD004366.

Sifferlin, A. (2013, October 16). Just Say No: When It Makes Sense Not to Take Your Medicine. *Time.* Retrieved from http://healthland.time.com/2013/10/16/just-say-no-when-it-makes-sense-not-to-take-your-medicine/

Smith, R. (2013). Introduction. In Peter C. Gøtzsche. *Deadly Medicines and Organised Crime: How Big Pharma Has Corrupted Healthcare.* London, United Kingdom: Radcliffe Publishing House.

*Statistics and outlook for chronic myeloid leukemia (CML).* (n.d.). Cancer Research UK. Retrieved from http://www.cancerresearchuk.org/cancer-help/type/cml/treatment/statistics-and-outlook-for-chronic-myeloid-leukaemia#cml

Sultan, S., & Hynes, N. (2013, July). The Ugly Side of Statins, Systemic Appraisal of the Contemporary Un-Known Unknowns. *Open Journal of Endocrine and Metabolic Disease, 3*(3), 179–185. doi:10.4236/ojemd.2013.33025

Thompson, D. (2013, November 18). Some doctors challenge the new statin guidelines. *HealthDay.* Retrieved from http://consumer.healthday.com/general-health-information-16/misc-drugs-news-218/new-statin-guidelines-questioned-by-some-docs-682290.html

Union of Concerned Scientists. (2006, July 20). *FDA Scientists pressured to exclude, findings; scientists fear retaliation for voicing safety concerns.* Reported in Peter C. Gøtzsche. (2013). *Deadly Medicines and Organised Crime: How Big Pharma Has Corrupted Healthcare* (p. 110). London, United Kingdom: Radcliffe Publishing House.

Vagnini, F., & Fox, B. (2006, March). Preventing pharmaceutical-induced nutritional deficiencies. Report. *LifeExtension.* Retrieved from http://www.lef.org/magazine/mag2006/mar2006_report_drugs_02.htm

# Chapter 4

*A Brief History and Timeline.* (n.d.). Neurogenesis, Neur 401 Advanced Neruoscience. Retrieved from http://sites.lafayette.edu/neur401-sp10/what-is-neurogenesis/a-timeline-of-research-adult-mammalian-neurogenesis/

Alzheimer's and Brain Research Center/Alzheimer's Association. (2014, September 17). *What we know today.* Retrieved from: http://www.alz.org/researchcenter

Alzheimer's disease. (n.d.). Retrieved from Wikipedia http://en.wikipedia.org/wiki/Alzheimer%27s_disease

Bailey, R. (n.d.). Hippocampus. *Free Biology Newsletter.* Retrieved from http://biology.about.com/od/anatomy/p/hippocampus.htm

Bowman, G. L., Silbert, L. C., Howieson, D., et al. (2012, January 24). Nutrient biomarker patterns, cognitive function, and MRI measures of brain aging. *Neurology, 78*(4), 241–9. doi:10.1212/WNL.0b013e3182436598

*Brain Parts and Function.* (n.d.). Brain Health & Puzzles. Retrieved from http://www.brainhealthandpuzzles.com/brain_parts_function.html

Cherry, K. (n.d.). Structure of a Neuron. About.com. Psychology. Retrieved from http://psychology.about.com/od/biopsychology/ss/neuronanat_3.htm

Cherry, K. (n.d.). What Is a Neurotransmitter? About.com. Psychology. Retrieved from http://psychology.about.com/od/nindex/g/neurotransmitter.htm

Cherry, K. (n.d.). What Is a Synapse? About.com. Psychology. Retrieved from http://psychology.about.com/od/sindex/f/what-is-a-synapse.htm

Cossins, D. (2013, June 7). Human Adult Neurogenesis Revealed. *The Scientist.* Retrieved from http://www.the-scientist.com/?articles.view/articleNo/35902/title/Human-Adult-Neurogenesis-Revealed/

Dendrite. (n.d.). In *The Free Dictionary* online. Retrieved from http://www.thefreedictionary.com/dendrite

DesMaisons, K. (1998). *Potatoes Not Prozac.* New York, NY: Fireside Book, Simon & Shuster.

Eriksson, P. S., Perfilieva, E., Björk-Eriksson, T., et al. (1998). Neurogenesis in the adult hippocampus. *1998 Nature America, Inc.* Retrieved from http://medicine.nature.com. 1998 Nature America Inc.

Ernst, A., Kanar, A., Bernard, S., et al. (2014, February 27). Neurogenesis in the Striatum of the Adult Human Brain. *Cell online, 156*(5), 1072–83. doi:10.1016/j.cell.2014.01.044

Fallon, S. (2001). *Nourishing Traditions* (Rev. 2nd ed.). Washington, DC: NewTrends Publishing, Inc.

Glycation. (n.d.). Retrieved from Wikipedia: http://en.wikipedia.org/wiki/Glycation

Gould, E., Beylin, A., Tanapat, P., et al. (1999, March). Learning enhances adult neurogenesis in the hippocampal formation. *Nature Neuroscience, 2*(3), 260–265 Retrieved from http://www.ncbi.nlm.nih.gov/pubmed/10195219 doi:10.1038/6365

Gould, E., & Gross, C. (2002, February 1). Neurogenesis in Adult Mammals: Some Progress and Problems. *Journal of Neuroscience, 22*(3), 619–623. Retrieved from http://www.jneurosci.org/content/22/3/619.full

Hillman, C. H., Erickson, K. L, & Kramer, A. F. (2008, January 9). Be smart, exercise your heart: Exercise effects on brain and cognition. *Nature Reviews Neuroscience, 9*(1), 58–65. Retrieved from http://www.ncbi.nlm.nih.gov/pubmed/18094706

Holford, P. (2007). *New Optimum Nutrition for the Brain.* United Kingdom: Piatkus Books Ltd.

Hurd, M., Martorell P., Delavande A., et al. (2013, April 4). Monetary Costs of Dementia in the United States. *New England Journal of Medicine, 368*(14), 1326–1334. doi:10.1056/NEJMsa1204629

Hyman, M. (2009). *The UltraMind Solution: Fix Your Broken Brain by Healing Your Body First.* New York, NY: Scribner.

Jesberger, J. A., & Richardson, J. S. (1991, March). Oxygen, Free Radicals and Brain Dysfunction. *International Journal of Neurosci*ence, *57*(1–2), 1–17. Retrieved from http://www.ncbi.nlm.nih.gov/pubmed/1938149

Juelich, F. (2013, October 10). New theory of synapse formation in the brain. *ScienceDaily.* Retrieved from http://www.sciencedaily.com/releases/2013/10/131010205325.htm

Kharrazian, D. (2013). *Why Isn't My Brain Working?* Carlsbad, CA: Elephant Press LP.

Kolb, B., & Whishaw, Q. (1998, February). Brain plasticity and behavior. *Annual Review of Psychology, 49*, 43–64. doi:10.1146/annurev.psych.49.1.43

Kramer A. F., & Ericson, K. I. (2007, August). Capitalizing on cortical plasticity: Influence of physical activity on cognition and brain function. *Trends in Cognitive Science, 11*(8): 342–8. Retrieved from http://www.ncbi.nlm.nih.gov/pubmed/17629545

Lindeberg, S. (2010). *Food and Western Disease: Health and Nutrition from an Evolutionary Perspective.* Chichester, West Sussex: John Wiley & Sons Ltd.

Logan, A. C. (2007). *The Brain Diet*. Nashville, TN: Cumberland House Publishing.

Myelin. (n.d.). *MedlinePlus Medical Encyclopedia*. Retrieved from www.nlm.nih.gov/medlineplus/ency/article/002261.htm

Myers, C. E. (2010, Winter). Glossary: Free radical. *The Newletter of the Memory Disorders Project at Rutgers University*.

Neuroplasticity. (n.d.). Retrieved from Wikipedia: http://en.wikipedia.org/wiki/Neuroplasticity

*Newborn Neurons Abundant in Adult Human Hippocampus*. (n.d.). Alzforum. Retrieved from http://www.alzforum.org/news/research-news/newborn-neurons-abundant-adult-human-hippocampus

Ono, K., Hamaguchi, T., Naiki, H., et al. (2006, June). Anti-amyloidogenic effects of antioxidants: Implications for the prevention and therapeutics of Alzheimer's disease. *BBA—Molecular Basis of Disease, 176*(6), 575–586. doi.org/10.1016/j.bbadis.2006.03.002

Ono, K., & Yamada, M. (2012, April). Vitamin A and Alzheimer's disease. *Geriatrics & Gerontology International, 12*(2), 180–8. doi:10.1111/j.1447-0594.2011.00786.x

Ornstein, R., & Thompson, R. (1984). *The Amazing Brain*. Boston, MA: Houghton Mifflin Co.

*Protect—Heavy Metals*. (2004). Resources for Science Learning. The Franklin Institute. Retrieved from http://learn.fi.edu/learn/brain/metals.html

Purves, D., Augustine, G. J., Fitzpatrick, D., et al. (Eds.). (2001). *Neuroscience* (2nd ed.). Sunderland, MA: Sinauer Associates. Retrieved from http://www.ncbi.nlm.nih.gov/books/NBK10799/

Sadli, N., Ackland, M. L., DeMel, D., et al. (2012). Effects of Zinc and DHA on the Epigenetic Regulation of Human Neuronal Cells. *Cell Physiology Biochemistry, 29*(1–2), 87–98. doi:10.1159/000337590

Schmidt, M. A. (2007). *Brain-Building Nutrition: How Dietary Fats and Oils Affect Mental, Physical, and Emotional Intelligence* (3rd ed.). Berkeley, CA: Frog Books Ltd.

Tan, Z. S., Harris, W. S., Beiser, A. S., et al. (2012, February 28). Red blood cell omega-3 fatty acid levels and markers of accelerated brain aging. *Neurology, 78*(9), 658–64. doi:10.1212/WNL.0b013e318249f6a9

Tangney, C. C., Tangney, N. T., Aggarwal, H., et al. (2011, September 27). Vitamin B12, cognition, and brain MRI measures: A cross-sectional examination.

*Neurology, 77*(13), 1276–82. Retrieved from http://www.natap.org/2011/HIV/Neurology-2011-Tangney-1276-82.pdf

*The Biology Project*. (2003, September 30). University of Arizona Department of Biochemistry and Biophysics. Retrieved from www.biology.arizona.edu

The Endocrine System. (n.d.). Leaving Certificate Biology. Retrieved from http://leavingbio.net/endocrine%20system/endocrine%20system.htm

*The Neurogenesis Research Newsletter*. (n.d.). Retrieved from http://neurogenesisresearch.com/

Zimmer, C. (2014, February). Secrets of the brain. *National Geographic Magazine, 225*(2), 30–57.

# Chapter 5

*Alcohol and Leaky Gut Syndrome*. (n.d.). DARA Thailand Drug & Alcohol Rehabilitation Asia. Retrieved from http://alcoholrehab.com/alcohol-rehab/alcohol-and-leaky-gut-syndrome/

An altered gut microbiota can predict diabetes. (2013, June 13). *ScienceDaily*. Retrieved from http://www.sciencedaily.com/releases/2013/06/130603092328.htm

APT. (n.d.). Biology-Online.org, dictionary. Retrieved from http://www.biology.online.org/dictionary/Atp

Bailey, M. (2011). Exposure to a social stressor alters the structure of the intestinal microbiota: Implications for stressor-induced immunomodulation. *Brain, Behavior, and Immunity, 25*(3), 397. doi:10.1016/j.bbi.2010.10.023

Bailey, R. (2011). Digestive System: Nutrient Absorption. About.com. Biology. Retrieved from http://biology.about.com/od/organsystems/a/aa032107a.htm

Bailey, R. (n.d.). Ribosomes. About.com. Biology. Retrieved from http://biology.about.com/od/cellanatomy/p/ribosomes.htm

Bravo, J. (2011). *Ingestion of* Lactobacillus *strain regulates emotional behavior and central GABA receptor expression in a mouse via the vagus nerve*. Proceedings of the National Academy of Sciences of the United States of America. doi:10.1073/pnas.1102999108

Cabot, S. (n.d.). *Liver Doctor: Love Your liver and Live Longer*. Retrieved from http://www.liverdoctor.com/liver-problems/leaky-gut-syndrome

Campbell-McBride, N. (2014, January 28). A new approach to children's health, fussiness and digestion [Webinar]. In The Future of Nutrition Conference (January 27–31). The Institute for the Psychology of Eating.

Celiac Disease. (n.d.) *The Merck Manual Home Health Handbook for Patients & Caregivers*. Retrieved from www.merckmanuals.com/home/disorders_of_nutrition

Drossman, D., & Swantkowski, M. (n.d.). *History of Functional Disorders*. Center for Functional GI & Motility Disorders. Retrieved from www.med.unc.edu/IBS

*Epilepsy: Vagus Nerve Stimulation*. (n.d.). WebMD. Retrieved from www.webmd. com/epilepsy/guide/vagus-nerve-stimulation-vns

Everhart J. E. (Ed.). (2008). *The Burden of Digestive Diseases in the United States*. Bethesda, MD: National Institute of Diabetes and Digestive and Kidney Diseases, US Department of Health and Human Services. Retrieved from http://www.niddk.nih.gov/about-niddk/strategic-plans-reports/Pages/burden-digestive-diseases-united-states.aspx

Fungal Infections (Candida). (n.d.). *LifeExtension*. Retrieved from http://www.lef.org/protocols/infections/fungal_infections_Candida_01htm

Gershon, M. (1998). *The Second Brain*. New York: HarperCollins.

Human microbiome. (n.d.). Retrieved from Wikipedia: http://en.wikipedia.org/wiki/Human_microbiome

Hurley, D. (2011, December) Your Backup Brain. *Psychology Today*. p. 80–86.

Hyman, M. (2012). *The Blood Sugar Solution*. New York, NY: Little Brown & Co., Hachette Book Group.

Iliades, D. (n.d.). *Surprising Benefits of High-Fiber Foods*. Everyday Health. Retrieved from http://www.everydayhealth.com/health-report/nutrition/surprising-benefits-of-a-high-fiber-diet.aspx

Junger, A. (2013). *Clean Gut: The Breakthrough Plan for Eliminating the Root Cause of Disease and Revolutionizing Your Health*. New York, NY: HarperCollins Publishers.

Kharrazian, D. (2013). *Why Isn't My Brain Working?* Carlsbad, CA: Elephant Press LP.

LaPine, T. (2009, May 27–30). *The Gut-Brain Connection—An Inside Look at Depression* [Symposium]. Institute of Functional Medicine, Hollywood, FL.

Larsen N., Vogensen, F. K., Van den Berg, F., et al. (2012, February 5). Gut Microbiota in Human Adults with Type 2 Diabetes Differs from Non-Diabetic Adults. *PLOS One*, 5(2), 9085. doi:10.1371/journal.pone.0009085

Lipski, E. (2012). *Digestive Wellness*, (4th ed.). San Francisco: McGraw-Hill.

Microbiome. (n.d.). Retrieved from Wikipedia: http://en.wikipedia.org/wiki/Microbiome

Mitochondria. (n.d.). Hyperphysics. Georgia State University. Retrieved from http:// hyperphysics.phy-astr.gsu.edu/hbase/biology/mitochondria.html

*Opportunities & Challenges in Digestive Diseases Research: Recommendations of the National Commission on Digestive Diseases.* (2009). National Institutes of Health, US Department of Health and Human Services. Bethesda, MD: National Institutes of Health. NIH Publication 08-6514.

Portal-vein. (n.d.). *Encyclopedia Britannica online.* Retrieved from http://www. britannica.com/EBchecked topic/471037/portal-vein

Proctor, L. (2012, February 22). Defining the Human Microbiome. A Food Forum Workshop on the Human Microbiome, Diet and Health. Institute of Medicine of the National Academy. Retrieved from http://www.ncbi.nlm.nih.gov/books/ NBK154092/

*The Gut Microbiome—The Future of Research & Patient Care* [video]. (n.d.). American Gastroenterological Association. AGA Congressional briefing. Retrieved from http:// www.gastro.org/advocacy-regulation/regulatory-issues/fecal-microbiota-transplant/ the-gut-microbiome-the-future-of-research-and-patient-care

*Vagus nerve stimulation.* (n.d.). Mayo Clinic. Retrieved from MayoClinic.com. www. mayoclinic.com/health/vagus-nerve-stimulation/MY00183

Watson, B., & Smith, L. (2003). *Gut Solutions: Natural Solutions to Your Digestive Problems.* Clearwater, FL: Renew Life Press and Information Services.

Wilhelmsen, I. (2000). Brain-gut axis as an example of the bio-psycho-social model. *Gut, 47*(Suppl IV), iv5–iv7. doi:10.1136/gut.47.suppl_4.iv5

Woolston, C. (n.d.). *Gut feelings: The surprising link between mood and digestion.* Consumer Health Interactive. Retrieved from www.ahealthyme.com/ article/primer/101186767

# Chapter 6

A reason to avoid this common chemical. (2010, September 8). Men's Health: The Doctors Health Press Editorial Board. *The Doctors Health Press.* Retrieved from www.doctorshealthpress.com

Beck, M. (2011, March 15). Clues to Gluten Sensitivity. Life and Culture. *Wall Street Journal.* Retrieved from http://online.wsj.com/news/articles/SB10001424 05274870489360457620039352245663

Beydoun, M. A., Beydoun, H. A., & Yang, Y. (2008, May). Obesity and central obesity as risk factors for incident dementia and its subtypes: a systematic review and meta-analysis. *Obesity Review, 9*(3), 204–18. Retrieved from doi:10.1111/ j.1467-789X. 2008.00473.x

Calderon-Garciduenas, L. (2004). Brain inflammation and Alzheimer's-like pathology in individuals exposed to severe air pollution. *Toxicologic, 32,* 650–658. Retrieved from http://tpx.sagepub.com/content/32/6/650.short

Challem, J. (2010). *The Inflammation Syndrome.* Hoboken, NJ: John Wiley & Sons, Inc.

Cox, J. (2013, August/September). Roundup Unready. *Organic Gardening Magazine.* Retrieved from http://www.organicgardening.com/living/roundup-unready

Davis, J. (n.d.). *How antioxidants work.* WebMD. Retrieved from www.webmd.com/ food-recipes/features/how-antioxidants-work1

Fife, B. (2011). *Stop Alzheimer's Now!* Colorado Springs, CO: Piccadilly Press.

*Food allergies: understanding food labels.* (2011, April 1). Mayo Clinic. Retrieved from http://www.mayoclinic.org/diseases-conditions/food-allergy/in-depth/ food-allergies/ART-20045949

Gerth, J., & Miller, T. (2013, September 20). Overdose: Use Only as Directed. *Propublica.* Retrieved from http://www.propublica.org/article/ tylenol-mcneil-fda-use-only-as-directed

Gittleman, A. (2010). *Zapped.* New York: HarperCollins.

Gittleman, A. L. (2012, March 16–18). *Your Home, Your Health: How to Make a Supernatural Sanctuary for Optimum Healing and Blood Sugar Balance.* Presentation given at the Nutritional Therapy Association annual conference. Vancouver, WA.

Hugo, E. R., Brandebourg, T. D., Woo, J. G., et al. (2008, December). Bisphenol A at environmentally relevant doses inhibits adiponectin release from human adipose tissue explants and adipocytes. *Environmental Health Perspectives, 116*(12), 1642–1647. Retrieved from http://www.ncbi.nlm.nih.gov/pubmed/19079714

*Is Oxidation Harmful Or Beneficial To Human Beings?* (n.d.). Wise Dude. Retrieved from http://www.wisedude.com/health_medicine/oxidation.htm

Jesberger J. A., & Richardson, J. S. (1991, March). Oxygen Free Radicals and Brain Dysfunction. *International Journal of Neuroscience, 57*(1–2), 1–17. Retrieved from http://informahealthcare.com/doi/abs/10.3109/00207459109150342

Kamer, A. R., Craig, R. G., & Dasanayake, A. P. (2008). Inflammation and Alzheimer's disease: Possible role of periodontal disease [Data file]. *Elsevier.* Retrieved from http://www.pharmaden.net/pdf/articles/22.pdf

Kolbert, E. (2010, November 24). A Warning by Key Researcher on Risks of BPA in Our Lives. *Yale Environment 360*. Retrieved from http://e360.yale.edu/feature/a_warning_by_key_researcher_on_risks_of_bpa_in_our_lives/2344/

Kolbert, E. (2012, February/2012, March). Is there poison in our food? Concerns about BPA. *Mother Earth News* (Green Gazette). Retrieved from http://www.motherearthnews.com/natural-health/bpa-zmgz12fmzrog.aspx#axzz3ADb3aZhm

Kristof, N. (2012, April 4). Arsenic in Our Chicken? *The New York Times*. Retrieved from http://www.nytimes.com/2012/04/05/opinion/kristof-arsenic-in-our-chicken.html?_r=0

Lean, G. (2008, June 29). US issues health warning over mercury fillings. *The Independent*. Retrieved from http://www.indepenent.co.uk/life-style/health-and-families-news/us-issues-health-warnings

Lindeberg, S. (2010). *Food and Western Disease: Health and Nutrition from an Evolutionary Perspective*. Chichester, West Sussex: John Wiley & Sons Ltd.

Miklossy, J. (2011, August 4). Alzheimer's disease—a neurospirochetosis. Analysis of the evidence following Koch's and Hill's criteria. *Journal of Neurinflammation*, *8*(90). doi:10.1186/1742-2094-8-90

Myers, C. E. (2010, Winter). Glossary: Free radical. In a newsletter of the memory disorders project at Rutgers University [Data file]. Retrieved from http://zung.zetamu.net/Library/Education/Education_Neuroscience/Gluck_Learning_and_Memory_2007.pdf

Palmer, C. (2012, August 30). Prevalence of periodontitis. *American Dental Association News*. Retrieved from www.ada.org/news/7543.aspx

Park, A. (2010, February 22). How to live to 100 years. *Time*, p. 56–66. Retrieved from http://www.pearsonhighered.com/assets/hip/us/hip_us_pearsonhighered/samplechapter/0205727646.pdf

Perlmutter, D. (2014, January 27). An Interview with Dr. David Perlmutter: *Grain Brain*. The Future of Nutrition Conference. Retrieved from http://experiencelife.com/newsflashes/free-online-event-the-future-of-nutrition-conference/

Pick, M. (n.d.). *An integrative approach to explaining systemic or chronic inflammation and its significance to your health*. Women to Women. Retrieved from www.womentowomen.com/inflammation/whatischronicinflammation.aspx

Pierini, C. (n.d.). Lectins: Their Damaging Role in Intestinal Health, Rheumatoid

Arthritis and Weight Loss. Vitamin Research Products. Retrieved from www.
vrp.com/digestive-health/lectins-their-damaging-role-in-intestinal-health

Reducing the threat of mercury. (2012, August/September). *National Wildlife*
(World Edition), p. 44.

Sapone, A., Lammers, K., Casolaro, V., et al. (2011, May 9). Divergence of gut
permeability and mucosal immune gene expression in two gluten-associated
conditions: celiac disease and gluten sensitivity. *BMC Medicine, 9*(32).
doi:10.1186/1741-7015-9-23

Scotti, K. (2008, January 19). *The dirty dozen—12 foods/food to avoid and why.* Food
Democracy. Retrieved from http://fooddemocracy.wordpress.com/2008/01/18/
the-dirty-dozen-12-foodsfood-additives-to-avoid-and-why/

Sullivan, K. (2012, February 7). *The Lectin Report.* Retrieved from www.krispin.
com/lectin.html

Turcotte, M. (2011, May 7). List of most inflammatory foods. Retrieved
from www.livestrong.com/article/30004-list-inflammatory-foods/

# Chapter 7

Ahlberg, A. C., Ljung, T., Rosmond R., et al. (2002, October 10). Depression and
anxiety symptoms in relation to anthropometry and metabolism in men. *Psychiatry Research, 2*(112), 101–10. Retrieved from http://www.ncbi.nlm.nih.gov/
pubmed/12429356

*Are all fats the same?* (n.d.). Spectrum Kitchen Guide. Retrieved from http://www.
spectrumorganics.com/images/uploads/496241e655274.pdf

Bazzano, L. A., Hu, T., Reynolds, K., et al. (2014, September 2). Effects of
low-carbohydrate and low fat diets: a randomized trial. *Annals of Internal Medicine, 161*(5), 309–318. doi: 10.7326/M14-0180

Boden-Albala, B., Elkind, M., White, H., et al. (2009, April). Dietary Total Fat
Intake and Ischemic Stroke Risk: The Northern Manhattan Study. *Neuroepide-
miology, 32*(4), 296–301. doi:10.1159/000204914

Buydens-Branchey, L., & Branchey, M. (2012, January 7). Long-chain n-3 polyunsaturated fatty acids decrease feeling of anger in substance abusers. *Psychiatry
Research, 157*(1–3), 95–104. Retrieved from http://www.sciencedirect.com/
science/article/pii/S0165178107000066

Campos, H., Blijlevens, E., McNamara, J. M., et al. (1992, December). LDL particles size distribution: Results from the Framingham Offspring Study. *Arteriosclerosis and Thrombosis: A Journal of Vascular Biology/American Heart Association, 12*(12), 1410–9. Retrieved from http://www.researchgate.net/ publication/21705893_LDL_particle_size_distribution._Results_from_the_ Framingham_Offspring_Study

ChooseMyPlate.gov. (n.d.). USDA. Retrieved from http://www.choosemyplate.gov/

*Cooking oils and smoke points in your kitchen.* (2010, April 27). The Culinary Works. Retrieved from http://www.theculinaryworks.com/index.php/ cooking-technique/foodie-facts/248-cooking-oils-and-smoke-points

Danaei, G., Ding, E. L., & Mozaffarian, D. (2009, April 28). The Preventable Causes of Death in the United States: Comparative Risk Assessment of Dietary, Lifestyle and Metabolic Risk Factors. *PLOS Medicine.* doi:10.1371/journal. pmed.1000058

*Dietary Guidelines for Americans 2005.* (n.d.). Chapter 6, Fats, Overview. Retrieved from http://www.health.gov/dietaryguidelines/dga2005/document/html/ chapter6.htm

Enig, M. G., & Fallon, S. (2000, January 1). *The Skinny on Fats.* The Weston A. Price Foundation. Retrieved from http://www.westonaprice.org/health-topics/ the-skinny-on-fats/

Estruch, R., Ros, E., Salas-Salvado, J., et al. (2013, April 4). Primary Prevention of Cardiovascular Disease with a Mediterranean Diet. *New England Journal of Medicine, 368*, 1279–1290. doi:10.1056/NEJMoa1200303

Fallon, S. (2001). *Nourishing Traditions* (Rev. 2nd ed.). Washington, DC: New Trends Publishing, Inc.

Gillman, M. W., Cupples L. A., Millen, B. E., et al. (1997, December 24–31). Inverse association of dietary fat with development of ischemic stroke in men. *The Journal of the American Medical Association, 278*(24), 2145–50. Retrieved from http://www.ncbi.nlm.nih.gov/pubmed/9417007

Gogos, C. A., Finopoulous, P., Salsa, B., et al. (1998, January 15). Dietary omega-3 polyunsaturated fatty acids plus vitamin E restore immunodeficiency and prolong survival for severely ill patients with generalized malignancy. *Cancer, 82*, 395–402. Retrieved from http://www.mccordresearch.com/sites/default/files/ research/Omega3_Immunodeficiency.pdf

Gordon, G., & Joiner-Bey, H. (2006). *The Omega-3 Miracle.* Topanga, CA: Freedom Press.

Herber, H., Feinleib, M., Mcnamara, P. M., & Castelli, W. P. (1983, May). Obesity as an Independent Risk Factor for Cardiovascular Disease: A 26-year Follow-Up of Participants in the Framingham Heart Study. *Circulation, 67*(5), 968–77. Retrieved from http://www.ncbi.nlm.nih.gov/pubmed/6219830

Hibbeln, J. R., & Salem, Jr., N. (1995, July). Dietary polyunsaturated fatty acids and depression: when cholesterol does not satisfy. *The American Journal of Clinical Nutrition, 62*, 1–9. Retrieved from http://ajcn.nutrition.org/content/62/1/1

Houston, M. (2012). *What Your Doctor May Not Tell You about Heart Disease.* New York: Grand Central Life & Style.

*How safe are fish oil supplements?* (2011). Environmental Defense Fund. Retrieved from Oceansalive.org/eat.cfm

Hu, Y., Block, G., Norkus, E. P., et al. (2006). Relations of glycemic index and glycemic load with plasma oxidative stress markers. *The American Journal of Clinical Nutrition, 84*(1), 70–76. Retrieved from http://ajcn.nutrition.org/content/84/1/70.full

Hyman, M. (2009). *The UltraMind Solution–Fix Your Broken Brain by Healing Your Body First.* York, NY: Schribner.

Irving, C. B., Mumby-Croft, M. F., & Joy, L. A. (2006, July 19). Polyunsaturated fatty acid supplementation for schizophrenia. *The Cochrane Library.* doi:10.1002/14651858.CD001257.pub2

Joy, C. B., Mumby-Croft, R., & Joy, L. A. (2003). Polyunsaturated fatty acid (fish or evening primrose oil) for schizophrenia. *Cochrane Database System Rev, 2003*(2), CD001257. PMID: 10796622

Kessler, R. C., Chiu, W. T., Demler, O., et al. (2005, June). Prevalence, severity, and comorbidity of twelve-month DSM-IV disorders in the National Comorbidity Survey Replication (NCS-R). *Archives of General Psychiatry, 62*, 617–27. Retrieved from http://www.ncbi.nlm.nih.gov/pubmed/15939839

Kharrazian, D. (2013). *Why Isn't My Brain Working?* Carlsbad, CA: Elephant Press LP.

Kris-Etherton, P., Harris, W., & Appel, L. (2002). Fish consumption, fish oil, omega-3 fatty acids and cardiovascular disease. *Circulation, 106*, 2747–2757. The American Heart Association, AHA Scientific Statement. doi:10.1161/01.CIR.0000038493.65177.94

Leas, C. (2008). *Fat: It's Not What You Think.* Amherst, NY: Prometheus Press.

Lin, P. Y., Huang, S. Y., & Su, K. P. (2010). A Meta-Analytic Review of Polyunsaturated Fatty Acid Compositions in Patients with Depression. *Biological*

*Psychiatry, 68*, 140–147. Retrieved from http://www.researchgate.net/ publication/44582651 A meta-analytic review of polyunsaturated fatty acid compositions in patients with depression

Lindeberg, S. (2010). *Food and Western Disease: Health and Nutrition from an Evolutionary Perspective*. Chichester, West Sussex: John Wiley & Sons Ltd.

Logan, A. C. (2007). *The Brain Diet*. Nashville, TN: Cumberland House Publishing.

Meydani, M., Natiello, F., Goldin, B., et al. (1990, August). Effect of Long-Term Fish Oil Supplementation on Vitamin E Status and Lipid Peroxidation in Women. *The Journal of Nutrition*. (Impact Factor: 4.2). 05/1991; *121*(4), 484-91. Retrieved from http://www.researchgate.net/publication/21330112 Effect of long-term fish oil supplementation on vitamin E status and lipid peroxidation in women

Monteiro, V. A. (2007, July–August). Dietary fat and ischemic stroke risk in Northern Portugal. *Acta Médica Portuguesa, 20*(4), 307–18. Retrieved from http://www.ncbi.nlm.nih.gov/pubmed/18198074

Muldoon, M. F., Ryan, C. M., Sheu, L., et al. (2010, February 24). Serum Phospholipid Docosahexaenonic Acid Is Associated with Cognitive Functioning During Middle Adulthood. *The Journal of Nutrition, 140*, 848–853. doi:10.3945/ jn.109.119578

Muller, T. (2012). *Extra Virginity: The Sublime and Scandalous World of Olive Oil*. New York, NY: W. W. Norton & Company, Inc.

Nair, P. P., Judd, J. T., Berlin, E., et al. (1993, July). Dietary fish oil-induced changes in the distribution of alpha-tocopherol, retinol, and beta-carotene in plasma, red blood cells, and platelets: modulation by vitamin E. *The American Journal of Clinical Nutrition, 58*(1), 98–102. Retrieved from http://ajcn.nutrition.org/ content/58/1/98.abstract

Nemets, H., Memets, B., Apter, A., et al. (2006, June). Omega-3 treatment of childhood depression. *American Journal of Psychiatry, 163*, 1098–1100. doi:10.1176/ appi.ajp.163.6.1098

Porro, J. (n.d.). *Cardiovascular Disease and the Endothelium* [Data file]. Breakthroughs in BioScience. Retrieved from www.faseb.org/portals/2/pdfs/opa/porro.pdf

Rondanelli, M., Giacosa, A., Opizzi, C., et al. (2011, January). Long chain omega-3 polyunsaturated fatty acids supplementation in the treatment of elderly depression: effects on depressive symptoms on the phospholipids fatty acid profile and on health-related quality of life. *The Journal of Nutrition, Health and Aging, 15*(1), 37–44. Retrieved from http://www.ncbi.nlm.nih.gov/pubmed/21267525

Sacks, F. (2010). *Ask the Nutrition Expert: Omega-3 Fatty Acids.* The Nutrition Source, Harvard School of Public Health. Retrieved from www.hsph.harvard.edu/nutritionsource/omega-eindes.html

Schmidt, M. A. (2007). *Brain-Building Nutrition: How Dietary Fats and Oils Affect Mental, Physical, and Emotional Intelligence* (3rd ed.). Berkeley, CA: Frog Books Ltd.

Severus, W., Ahrens, B., & Stoll, A. L. (1999, April). Omega-3 Fatty Acids: The Missing Link [Letter to the editor]. *Archives of General Psychiatry, 56,* 380–81. Retrieved from http://archpsyc.jamanetwork.com/issue.aspx?issueid=5085

Shaw, J. (2004). *Trans Fats: The Hidden Killer in Our Food.* New York, NY: Pocket Books.

Smith, R., & Pinckney, E. R. (1991). *Diet, Blood Cholesterol and Coronary Heart Disease: A Critical Review of the Literature, Vol 2.* Sherman Oaks, CA: Vector Enterprises.

Stoll, A. L. (2001). *The Omega-3 Connection.* New York, NY: Simon & Schuster.

Sublette, E. M., Hibbeln, J. R., Galfalvy, H. (2006). Omega-3 Polyunsaturated Essential Fatty Acid Status as a Predictor of Future Suicide Risk. *American Journal of Psychiatry. 163,* 1100–1102. doi:10.1176/appi.ajp.163.6.1100

Swerdlow, D. I., Holmes, M. V., & Kuchenbaecker, K. B. (2012, March 31). Interleukin-6 receptor pathways in coronary heart disease: a collaborative meta-analysis. *The Lancet, 379*(9822), 1214–1224. doi:10.1016/S0140-6736(12)60110-X

Van Gelder, B., Tijhuis, M., Kalmijn, S., & Kromhou, D. (2008, May 28). Fish consumption, n-C fatty acids, and subsequent decline in elderly men: the Zutphen Elderly Study. *The American Journal of Clinical Nutrition. 85,* 1142–1146. Retrieved from http://www.ncbi.nlm.nih.gov/pubmed/17413117

Voight, B., Peloso, G., Orho-Melander, M., et al. (2012, May 17). Plasma HDL cholesterol and risk of myocardial infarction: a mendelian randomisation study. *The Lancet, 380*(9841), 572–580. doi:10.1016/S0140-6736(12)60312-2

Walsh, B. (2014, June 23). Don't blame fat. *Time, 138*(24), 29–35.

Yaffe K., Kanaya, A., Lindquist, K., et al. (2004, November 11). The Metabolic Syndrome, Inflammation, and Risk of Cognitive Decline. *The Journal of the American Medical Association, 292*(18), 2237-42. doi:10.1001/jama.292.18.2237

# Chapter 8

Antinutrients—Your Key to Bad Health. (n.d.). Ben Balzer's Paleolithic Diet Site [Web blog]. Retrieved from http://paleolithicdiet.wordpress.com/2008/06/22/antinutrients-your-key-to-bad-health/

*Are Nuts and Seeds Healthy?* (2014, January 9). Paleo Diet Lifestyle. Retrieved from http://paleodietlifestyle.com/are-nuts-and-seeds-health

Belobrajdic, D. P., & Bird, A. R. (2013, May 16). The potential role of phytochemicals in whole grain cereals for the prevention of type-2 diabetes. *Nutrition Journal, 12*(62). doi:10.1186/1475-2891-12-62

Brooks, M. (2012, October 19). *High-Carb Diet May Raise Risk for Cognitive Impairment.* Medscape Medical News. Retrieved from http://www.medscape.com/viewarticle/772935

Crane, P., Walker, R., Hubbard, R. A., et al. (2013, August 8). Glucose Levels and Risk of Dementia. *New England Journal of Medicine, 369*(6), 540–8. doi:10.1056/NEJMoa1215740

*Dietary Fiber: Essential for a Healthy Diet.* (n.d.). Mayo Clinic Staff. Retrieved from http://www.mayoclinic.com/health/fiber/NU00033

*Eating more fiber may lower risk of first-time stroke.* (2013, March 28). American Heart Association. Retrieved from http://newsroom.heart.org/news/eating-more-fiber-may-lower-risk-of-first-time-stroke

Ellagic Acid. (n.d.). American Cancer Society. Retrieved from http://www.cancer.org/treatment/treatmentsandsideeffects/complementaryandalternativemedicine/dietandnutrition/ellagic-acid

Fallon, S. (1999). *Nourishing Traditions* (2nd ed.). Washington, DC: New Trends Publishing, Inc.

Finkelstein, E. A., Khavjou, O. A., Thompson, H., et al. (2012). Obesity and Severe Obesity Forecasts Through 2030. *American Journal of Preventive Medicine, 42*(6), 563–570. doi:10.1016/j.amepre.2011.10.026

Flavonoids. (n.d.). The World's Healthiest Foods. Retrieved from http://www.whfoods.com/genpage.php?tname=nutrient&dbid=119

*Gluten Free Whole Grains.* (n.d.). Whole Grains Council. Retrieved from http://www.wholegrainscouncil.org/whole-grains-101/gluten-free-whole-grains

Hadjivassiliou, M., Sanders, D. S., Grünewald, R. A., et al. (2010, March). Gluten

Sensitivity: from gut to brain. *Lancet Neurology, 9*(3), 318–30. doi:10.1016/S1474-4422(09)70290-X

Haffner, S. M., Liese, A. D., Haffner, S. M., et al. (2010, March). Whole and Refined Grain Intakes Are Related to Inflammatory Protein Concentrations in Human Plasma. *The Journal of Nutrition. 140*(3), 587–594. doi:10.002/hbm.20870

*High Fiber Food List for a High Fiber Diet.* (n.d.). CommonSenseHealth.com. Retrieved from http://www.commonsensehealth.com/Diet-and-Nutrition/List_of_High_Fiber_Foods.shtml

*How much sugar do you eat? You may be surprised!* [Data file]. (n.d.). New Hampshire Department of Health and Human Services, Division of Public Services Health, Promotion in Motion. Retrieved from http://www.dhhs.state.nh.us/dphs/nhp/adults/documents/sugar.pdf

*How Resveratrol May Fight Aging.* (2013, March 25). National Institutes of Health. Retrieved from http://www.nih.gov/researchmatters/march2013/03252013resveratrol.htm

Jean, L. (n.d.). Gluten Intolerance Symptoms—How Do You Know if Gluten is Making You Sick? *Gluten Free Network.* Retrieved from http://glutenfreenetwork.com/symptoms-treatments/gluten-intolerance-symptoms-how-do-you-know-if-gluten-is-making-you-sick/

Ji, S. (2013). The Critical Role of Wheat Lectin in Human Disease and the Role of Gluten in Cultural History and Consciousness [Webinar]. The Gluten Summit. Retrieved from www.greenmedinfo.com/gmi-blogs/sayer%20ji

Kaffashian, S., Dugravot, A., Elbaz, A., et al. (2013, April 2). Predicting cognitive decline. A dementia risk score vs the Framingham vascular risk scores. *Neurology, 80*(14), 1300–1306. doi:10.1212WNL.0b013e318ab370

Knopf, A. A. (n.d.). Ten Health Benefits of Fiber. *Forbes.* Retrieved from http://www.forbes.com/pictures/eikh45heid/weight-management/

Lefevre, M., & Jonnalagadda, S. (2012, July). Effect of Whole Grain on Markers of Subclinical Inflammation. *Nutrition Reviews, 70*(7). 387–96: doi:10.1111/j.1753-4887.2012. 00487.x

Lindeberg, S. (2010). *Food and Western Disease: Health and Nutrition from an Evolutionary Perspective.* Chichester, West Sussex: John Wiley & Sons Ltd.

Lund. E. (2003, March). Non-Nutritive Bioactive Constituents of Plants: Dietary and Health Benefits of Glucosinolates. *International Journal for Vitamin and Nutrition Research, 73*(2), 135–43. PMID: 12747221

Masters, R. C., Liese, A. D., Haffner, S. M., et al. (2010, March). Whole and refined grain intakes are related to inflammatory protein concentrations in human plasma. *The Journal of Nutrition, 140*(3), 587–594. doi:10.3945/jn.109.116640

Mercola, J. (2003). *The No-Grain Diet.* New York, NY: Plume, the Penguin Group.

Myers, A. (2013, May 6). *19 Foods That Cross-React With Gluten.* Primal Docs. Retrieved from http://primaldocs.com/opinion/19-foods-that-cross-react-with-gluten/

Nagel, R. (2010, March 26). *Living with Phytic Acid.* The Weston A. Price Foundation. Retrieved from http://www.westonaprice.org/food-features/living-phytic-acid

New research suggests choosing different fruits and vegetables may increase phytonutrient intake. (2010, April 26). *(e) Science News.* Retrieved from http://esciencenews.com/articles/2010/04/26/new.research.suggests.choosing.different.fruits.and.vegetables.may.increase.phytonutrient.intake

*Obese People Have "Severe Brain Degeneration."* (2009, August 25). LiveScience. Retrieved from www.livescience.com/10582-obese-people-have-severe-brain-degeneration.html/

Ornstein, R., & Sobel, D. (1987). *The Healing Brain.* New York, NY: Simon & Schuster.

Osborne, P. (2013, November). How Cross-Reactivity, Molecular Mimicry and Mold Toxicity Can Seriously Impact Your Health [Webinar]. The Gluten Summit. Retrieved from www.glutenfreesociety.org

*Overweight and Obesity in the U.S.* (n.d.). Food Research and Action Center. Retrieved from http://frac.org/initiatives/hunger-and-obesity/obesity-in-the-us/

Phytonutrient FAQs. (n.d.). United States Department of Agriculture. Agriculture Research Service. Retrieved from http://www.ars.usda.gov/aboutus/docs.htm?docid=4142

Raji, C. A., Ho, A. J., Parikshak, N., et al. (2010, March 3). Brain Structure and Obesity. *Human Brain Mapping, 31*(3), 353–64. doi:10.1002/hbm.20870

Roberts, R. O., Roberts, L. S., Geda, Y. E., et al. (2012). Relative Intake of Macro-nutrients Impacts Risk of Mild Cognitive Impairment of Dementia. *Journal of Alzheimer's Disease, 32*(2), 329–39. doi:10.3233/JAD-2012-120862

Ros, E. (2010, July). Health Benefits of Nut Consumption. *Nutrients, 2*(7), 652–82. Retrieved from http://www.ncbi.nlm.nih.gov/pmc/articles/PMC3257681/

Sabharwal, N. (2012, October 20). High-carb diet may impair mental function—study. TheMedGuru. *Medscape Medical News* > *Psychiatry*. Retrieved from http://www.themedguru.com/20121020/newsfeature/high-carb-diets-may-impair-mental-function—study-86147123.html

Taubes, G. (2011). *Why We Get Fat: And What to do About It*. New York: Anchor Books.

The Benefits of Soaking Nuts and Seeds. (n.d.). *Food Matters*. Retrieved from http://foodmatters.tv/articles-1/the-benefits-of-soaking-nuts-and-seeds

Walter, J., Martinez, I., & Rose D. J. (2013, July–August). Holobiont nutrition: Considering the role of gastrointestinal microbiota in the health benefits of whole grains. *Gut Microbes, 4*(4), 340–6. doi:10.4161/gmic.24707. … PMID: 23645316

*Weight Loss & Diet Plans: Phytonutrients*. (n.d.). WebMD. Retrieved from http://www.webmd.com/diet/phytonutrients-faq

Zelman, K. (n.d.). *The benefits of fiber: For your heart, weight, and energy. Dietary fiber: insoluble vs. insoluble.* WebMD. Retrieved from http://www.webmd.com/diet/fiber-health-benefits-11/insoluble-soluble-fiber

# Chapter 9

*Air quality*. (n.d.). Grace Communication Foundation Food Program. Retrieved from http://sustainabletable.org/266/air-quality

Amino Acids. (n.d.). *MedlinePlus Medical Encyclopedia*. Retrieved from http://www.nlm.nih.gov/medlineplus/ency/article/002222.htm

Bowden, J. (2013, May 1). Carnitine Confusion: What Does That New Red Meat Study Really Mean? *Huffpost Healthy Living*. Retrieved from http://www.huffingtonpost.com/dr-jonny-bowden/red-meat-health_b_3119520.html

Carlton, M., & Carlton, J. (2013). *Rich Food, Poor Food: The Ultimate Grocery Producing System (GPS)*. Malibu, CA: Primal Blueprint Publishing.

*Common Vegan Diet Deficiencies & Prevention Tips*. (n.d.). FitDay. Retrieved from http://www.fitday.com/fitness-articles/nutrition/healthy-eating/common-vegan-diet-deficiencies-prevention-tips.html

*Confused About Soy?—Soy Dangers Summarized*. (n.d.). The Weston A. Price Foundation. Retrieved from http://www.westonaprice.org/soy-alert/

Dash, P. (1997–present). *Neuroscience Online, an Electronic Textbook for the Neurosciences*. Chapter 11: Blood Brain Barrier and Cerebral Metabolism, Transport of Glucose and Amino Acids. The UT Medical School at Houston. Retrieved from http://neuroscience.uth.tmc.edu/s4/chapter11.html

Dolson, L. (2012, October 9). Low Carb Diets. List of high-protein food and amount of protein in each. About.com. Retrieved from http://lowcarbdiets.about.com/od/whattoeat/a/highproteinfood.htm

*Factory Farming and Human Health.* (n.d.). People for the Ethical Treatment of Animals (PETA). Retrieved from http://www.peta.org/issues/factory-farming-and-human-health.aspx

*Factory Farming and the Environment.* (n.d.). People for the Ethical Treatment of Animals (PETA). Retrieved from http://www.peta.org/issues/factory-farms-and-the-environment.aspx

Fallon, S. (2001). *Nourishing Traditions* (Rev. 2nd ed.). Washington, DC: New Trends Publishing, Inc.

German, J. B., Gibson, R. A., & Krauss, R. M. (2009, June). A reappraisal of the impact of dairy foods and milk fat on cardiovascular disease risk. *European Journal of Nutrition, 48*(4), 191–203. doi:10.1007/s00394-009-0002-5

Journel, M., Chaumontet, C., Darcel, N., et al. (2012, May). Brain Response to High

Koeth, R. A., Wang, Z., Levison, B. S., et al. (2013, April 7). Intestinal microbiota metabolism of L-carnitine, a nutrient in red meat, promotes atherosclerosis. *Nature Medicine, 19*, 576–585. doi:10.1038/nm.3145

Lindeberg, S. (2010). *Food and Western Disease: Health and Nutrition from an Evolutionary Perspective.* Chichester, West Sussex: John Wiley & Sons Ltd.

Ludwig D. S., & Willett, W. C. (2013, September) Three Daily Servings of Reduced-Fat Milk: An Evidence-Based Recommendation? *The Journal of the American Medical Association Pediatrics.* Accessed 2013, July 3. doi:10.1001/jamapediatrics.2013.2408

Micha, R., Wallace, S. K., & Mozaffarian, D. (2010, June 1,). Red and Processed Meat Consumption and Risk of Incident Coronary Heart Disease, Stroke and Diabetes: A Systematic Review and Meta-Analysis. *Circulation, 121*(21), 2271–2283. doi:10.1161/CirculationAHA.109.924977

Nachman, K. E., Baron, P. A., Raber, G., et al. (2013, July). Roxarsone, Inorganic Arsenic, and Other Arsenic Species in Chicken: A U.S.-Based Market Basket Sample. *Environmental Health Perspectives, 121*(7), 818–24. doi:10.1289/ehp.1206245

*Nutrition in Depth: What is a Protein?* (n.d.). Harvard School of Public Health.

Retrieved from The Nutrition Source: www.hsph.harvard.edu/nutritionsource/
what-should-you.../protein/

*Nutritional Protocol for Infants—Ages 0 – 2 years.* (n.d.). The National Association
for Child Development, Health & Nutrition. Retrieved from http://nacd.org/
health/protocol.php

Pan A., Sun, Q., Bernstein, A. M., et al. (2012, March 12). Red Meat Consumption
and Mortality: Results from 2 Prospective Cohort Studies. *Archives of Internal
Medicine, 172*(7), 555–563. doi:10.1001/archinternmed.2011.2287

Pawlak, R., Parrott, S. J., Raj S., et al. (2013, February). How prevalent is vitamin
B(12) deficiency among vegetarians? *Nutrition Review, 71*(2), 110–17.
doi:10.1111/nure.12001

Protein. (n.d.). Retrieved from Wikipedia: http://en.wikipedia.org/wiki/
protein-(nutrient)

Protein Diets. (n.d.). *Advanced Nutrition, 3,* 322–329. doi:10.3945/an.112.002071

*Raw Milk vs. Pasteurized Milk* (2013, November 21). Retrieved from http://www.
realmilk.com/health/raw-milk-vs-pasteurized-milk/

Soybeans. (n.d.). The World's Healthiest Foods. The George Mateljan
Foundation. Retrieved from http://www.whfoods.com/genpage.
php?tname=foodspice&dbid=79

*The Dangers of Raw Milk: Unpasteurized Milk Can Pose a Serious Health Risk.* (n.d.).
US Food and Drug Administration, Food Facts. Retrieved from http://www.
fda.gov/Food/ResourcesForYou/consumers/ucm079516.html

Thompson, D. (2013, August 28). *Brain Protein Is a Key to "Senior
Moments."* WebMD Brain & Nervous System Health Center.
Retrieved from http://www.webmd.com/brain/news/20130828/
brain-protein-is-a-key-to-senior-moments-study-finds

Vegetarian nutrition. (n.d.). Retrieved from Wikipedia: http://en.wikipedia.org/wiki/
Vegetarian_nutrition

*Vitamin B12 Deficiency Seen in All Types of Vegetarians.* (2003, June 18). WebMD.
Retrieved from http://www.webmd.com/food-recipes/news/20030618/
vegetarian-diet-b12-deficiency

Walsh, B. (2014, June 23). Don't blame fat. *Time,* p. 28–35.

Weber, K. (Editor). (2009). *Food, Inc.* [Documentary film]. Another Take: Food
Safety Consequences of Factory Farms. Food & Water Watch. New York, NY:
Public Affairs.

*Why You Need Protein in Your Diet.* (n.d.). For Dummies. Retrieved from http://www. dummies.com/how-to/content/why-you-need-protein-in-your-diet.html

Wiley (2013, August 22). Breast is best: Good bacteria arrive from mum's gut via breast milk. *ScienceDaily.* Retrieved from http://www. sciencedaily.com/releases/2013/08/130822091026.htm

# Chapter 10

Amen, D. J. (2011). *The Amen Solution.* New York, NY: Crown Archtype.

Arcidiacomo, B., Iiritano, S., Nocera, A., et al. (2012, April 10). Insulin Resistance and Cancer Risk: An Overview of the Pathogenic Mechanisms. *Journal of Diabetes Research.* Article ID 789174. Retrieved from http://www.hindawi.com/ journals/jdr/2012/789174/cta/

Artificial Sweeteners. (n.d.). MedicineNet. Retrieved from http://www.medicinenet. com/script/main/art.asp?articlekey=81475

Ashton, M. (2011). *Agave & Stevia Comparison.* Retrieved from http://www. livestrong.com/article/408618-agave-stevia-comparison

Baskin, D. G., Blevins, J. E., & Schwartz, M. W. (2001). How the brain regulates food intake and body weight: The role of leptin. *Journal of Pediatric Endocrinology Metabolism, 14*(Suppl 6), 1417–29. PMID:11837495

Brain atrophy linked with cognitive decline in diabetes. (2013, September 12). Monash University. *ScienceDaily.* Retrieved from www.sciencedaily.com/ releases/2013/09/130912093807.htm

Brody, J. (2013, February 16). Artificial Sweeteners—Times Topics. *The New York Times.* Retrieved from http://topics.nytimes.com/top/reference/timestopics/ subjects/s/sweeteners_artificial/index.html

*Child Obesity Facts.* (n.d.). Center for Disease Control and Prevention. Retrieved from http://www.cdc.gov/healthyyouth/obesity/facts.htm

Choose *MyPlate*, Food Groups. (n.d.). United State Department of Agriculture. Retrieved from www.choosemyplate.gov

Cohen, R. (2013, August). Sugar Love (A Not So Sweet Story). *National Geographic, 224*(3), 78–97.

De Koning, L., Malik, V. S., Kellogg, M. D., et al. (2012, March 12). Sweetened Beverage Consumption, Incident Coronary Heart Disease and Biomarkers of Risk in Men. *Circulation.* doi:10.1161/ CIRCULATIONAHA.111.067017

*Diabetes Basics*. (n.d.). American Diabetes Association. Retrieved from http:// www.diabetes.org/diabetes-basics/diabetes-statistics/

Does Sugar Feed Cancer? (2009, August 18). University of Utah Health Sciences. *ScienceDaily*. Retrieved from www.sciencedaily.com/ releases/2009/08/090817184539.htm

Dolson, L. (2008, May 2). Is the Glycemic Index useful? About.com. Low-carb diets. Retrieved from http://lowcarbdiets.about.com/od/nutrition/p/glycemicindex. html

Even in normal range, high blood sugar linked to brain shrinkage [Press release]. (2012, September 3). American Academy of Neurology. Retrieved from https:// www.aan.com/PressRoom/Home/PressRelease/1100

Excess sugar linked to cancer. (2013, February 1). Madrimasd. *ScienceDaily* Retrieved from http://www.sciencedaily.com/releases/2013/02/130201100149.htm

Fallon, S. (2001). *Nourishing Traditions* (Rev. 2nd ed.). Washington, DC: New Trends Publishing, Inc.

Godman, H. (2013, August 7). Above-normal blood sugar linked to dementia. *Harvard Health Letter*. Retrieved from http://www.health.harvard.edu/blog/ above-normal-blood-sugar-linked-to-dementia-201308076596

High fructose corn syrup. (n.d.). Retrieved from Wikipedia: http://en.wikipedia.org/ wiki/High_fructose_corn_syrup

Howard, B. V., & Wylie-Rosett, J. (2002). Sugar and Cardiovascular Disease. AHA Scientific Statement. *Circulation, 106*, 523-527. doi:10.1161/ 01.CIR.0000019552.77778.04

Hyman, M. (2012). *The Blood Sugar Solution*. New York, NY: Little Brown & Co., Hachette Book Group.

Jegvig, S. (2014, February, 11). Guess how much sugar in a can of cola. About.com. Nutrition. Retrieved from http://nutrition.about.com/od/ healthyappetizerssnacks/f/how-much-sugar-in-cola.htm

King, R. H. M. (2001). The role of glycation in the pathogenesis of diabetic polyneuropathy. *Molecular Pathology, 54*(6), 400–408. Retrieved from http://www.ncbi. nlm.nih.gov/pmc/articles/PMC1187130/

Kirkpatrick, K. (2013, July 30). 10 Things You Don't Know About Sugar (And What You Don't Want to Know Could Hurt You). *Huffpost Healthy Living*. Retrieved from http://www.huffingtonpost.com/kristin-kirkpatrick-ms-rd-ld/dangers-of-sugar_b_3658061.html

Kiyohara, Y. (2011, November). The cohort study of dementia: The Hisayama Study [Abstract]. *Rinsho Shinkeigaku, 51*(11), 906–909. Retrieved from http://www. ncbi.nlm.nih.gov/pubmed/22277412

Krieger, E. (2012, February 12). *The Scoop on Stevia*. Retrieved from http://www. elliekrieger.com/the-scoop-on-Stevia

Lactitol. (n.d.). Retrieved from Wikipedia: http://en.wikipedia.org/wiki/Lactitol

Larsson, S. C., Bergkvist, L., & Wolk, A. (2006, November). Consumption of sugar and sugar-sweetened foods and the risk of pancreatic cancer in a prospective study. *The American Journal of Clinical Nutrition, 84*(5), 1171–1176. Retrieved from http://ajcn.nutrition.org/content/84/5/1171.full

Lindeberg, S. (2010). *Food and Western Disease: Health and Nutrition from an Evolutionary Perspective*. Chichester, West Sussex: John Wiley & Sons Ltd.

*Lower blood sugars may be good for the brain*. (2013, October 23). American Academy of Neurology. Retrieved from http://www.sciencedaily.com/ releases/2013/10/131023165016.htm

Lustig, R. H. (2012, May 12). *The Diet Debacle*. Project Syndicate. Retrieved from http://www.project-syndicate.org/print/the-diet-debacle

Lustig, R. H., Schmidt, L. A., & Brindis, C. D. (2012, February 2). The toxic truth about sugar. Comment, *Nature, 482*, 27–29. Retrieved from http://www.paho. org/nutricionydesarrollo/wp-content/uploads/2012/05/Comment.-Toxic-truth-about-sugar.pdf

McCleary, L. (2011). *Feed Your Brain, Lose Your Belly*. Austin, TX: Greenleaf Book Group Press.

Mercola, J. (2006). *Sweet Deception: Why Splenda, NutraSweet, and the FDA May Be Hazardous to Your Health*. Nashville, TN: Thomas Nelson, Inc.

Norris, J. (2009, June 25). Sugar Is a Poison, Says UCSF Obesity Expert. *UCSF Magazine*. Retrieved from http://www.ucsf.edu/news/2009/06/8187/ obesity-and-metabolic-syndrome-driven-fructose-sugar-diet

*Overweight and Obesity*. (n.d.). Center for Disease Control and Prevention. Retrieved from http://www.cdc.gov/obesity/data/adult.html

Page, K. A., Chan, O., Arora, J., et al. (2013, January 2). Effects of Fructose vs. Glucose on Regional Cerebral Blood Flow in Brain Regions Involved With Appetite and Reward Pathways. *The Journal of the American Medical Association, 309*(1), 63–70. doi:10.1001/jama.2012.116975

Peeke, P. (2012). *The Hunger Fix: The Three-Stage Detox Recovery Plan for Overeating and Food Addiction.* New York, NY: Rodale Press.

Perlmutter, D. (2013). *Grain Brain.* New York, NY: Little Brown and Company, Hachette Book Group.

Richards, B. (2009). *Mastering Leptin* (3ʳᵈ ed.). Minneapolis, MN: Wellness Resource Books.

Roberts, H. J. (2001). *Aspartame Disease: An Ignored Epidemic.* West Palm Beach, FL: Sunshine Sentinel Press.

Schardt, D. (2008, October). Stevia, Sweet … but How Safe? [Data file]. *Nutrition Action Healthletter.* Retrieved from http://cspinet.org/new/pdf/stevia_update.pdf

Seely S., & Horrobin, D. F. (1983, July). Diet and breast cancer: The possible connection with sugar consumption. *Medical Hypotheses, 11*(3), 319–327. Retrieved from http://www.ncbi.nlm.nih.gov/pubmed/6645999

Sisson, M. (2010, June 17). *A Primal Primer: Leptin.* Mark's Daily Apple. Retrieved from www.marksdailyapple.com/leptin/#azxx28MVUPXQQ

*Sugar overload can damage heart according to UTHealth research.* (2013, June 14). University of Texas, Health Science Center of Houston. Retrieved from https://www.uth.edu/media/story.htm?id=020d26f7-c04e-43c3-94a9-1fc4110ef2a7

Sugar Substitutes. (n.d.). Retrieved from Wikipedia: http://en.wikipedia.org/wiki/Sugar_substitute

Taubes, G. (2011, April 13). An interview with C. Thompson in Is Sugar Toxic? *The New York Times.* Retrieved from http://www.nytimes.com/2011/04/17/magazine/mag-17Sugar-t.html?pagewanted=all

This Sweetener Is Far Worse Than High Fructose Corn Syrup. (2010, April 15). *Huffpost Healthy Living.* Retrieved from www.huffingtonpost.com/dr.../agave-this-sweetener-is-f_b_537936.html

*Too Much Sugar Can Cause Heart Failure.* (2013, June 13). Medical News Today. Retrieved from http://www.medicalnewstoday.com/articles/262014.php

Top 4 Most Dangerous Artificial Sweeteners. (n.d.) *FitDay.* Retrieved from http://www.fitday.com/fitness-articles/nutrition/healthy-eating/top-number-most-dangerous-artificial-sweeteners.html#b

Top 5 Healthiest Natural Sweeteners. (n.d.). *FitDay.* Retrieved from http://www.fitday.com/fitness-articles/nutrition/healthy-eating/top-5-healthiest-natural-sweeteners.html#b

Tudor, A. (2012). *Sweet Potato Power: Smart Carbs; Paleo and Personalized.* Las Vegas, NV: Victoria Belt Publishing Co.

Walton, A. G. (2013, November 23). Sugary Drinks Linked to Cancer Risk in Women. Pharm & HealthCare. *Forbes.* Retrieved from http://www.forbes.com/ sites/alicegwalton/2013/11/23/sugary-drinks-linked-to-cancer-risk-in-women/

Wiley, S. S. (2013, October 26). *Obesity History in America.* Livestrong.com. Retrieved from http://www.livestrong.com/ article/359624-obesity-history-in-america/

Yang, Q., Zhang, Z., Gregg, E. W., et al. (2014, February). Added Sugar Intake and Cardiovascular Diseases Mortality Among US Adults. *The Journal of the American Medical Association Internal Medicine.* Retrieved from doi:10.1001/jamainternmed.2013.13563

# Chapter 11

Adults worldwide eat almost double daily AHA recommended amount of sodium. (2013, March 21). American Heart Association Report. Retrieved from http:// newsroom.heart.org/news/adults-worldwide-eat-almost-double-daily-aha-recommended-amount-of-sodium

Alcohol's Damaging Effects on the Brain. (2004). National Institute on Alcohol and Abuse. *Alcohol Alert, Number 63.* Retrieved from http://pubs.niaaa.nih.gov/ publications/aa63/aa63.htm

American Council on Exercise. (n.d.) Fit Facts. Healthy Dydration [Data file]. Retrieved from http://www.acefitness.org/fitfacts/pdfs/fitfacts/itemid_173.pdf

Amour, S. (2013, March 21). High Salt Consumption Tied to 2.3 Million Heart Deaths. *Bloomberg.* Retrieved from http://www.bloomberg.com/news/2013-03-21/high-salt-consumption-tied-to-2-3-million-heart-deaths.html

Boesler, M. (2013, July). You Are Paying 300 Times More for Bottled Water than Tap Water. Business Insider. *Slate Magazine.* Retrieved from http://www.slate. com/blogs/business_insider/2013/07/12/cost_of_bottled_water_vs_tap_water_ the_difference_will_shock_you.html

*Bottled Water: Pure Drink or Pure Hype?* (2013, July). National Resources Defense Council. Retrieved from http://www.nrdc.org/water/drinking/bw/bwinx.asp

Brody, J. (2013, April 19). People who have less salt in their diet live healthier, longer.

*Deccan Herald.* Retrieved from http://www.deccanherald.com/content/324770/people-have-less-salt-their.html

Brownstein, D. (2006). *Salt Your Way to Health.* West Bloomfield, MI: Medical Alternative Press.

*Commercially Bottled Water.* (2014, April). Center for Disease Control. Retrieved from http://www.cdc.gov/healthywater/drinking/bottled/

Edgar, J. (2009, March 20). *Types of Teas and Their Benefits.* WebMD. Retrieved from http://www.webmd.com/diet/features/tea-types-and-their-health-benefits

*Energy Drink Consumption Now a Serious Public Health Threat.* (2013, January). Medical News Today. Retrieved from http://www.medicalnewstoday.com/articles/255078.php

Epigallocatechin gallate. (n.d.). Retrieved from Wikipedia: http://en.wikipedia.org/wiki/Epigallocatechin_gallate#Pharmacology

Goodman, S. (2009, July). Fewer Regulations for Bottled Water Than Tap, GAO says. *The New York Times.* Retrieved from http://www.nytimes.com/gwire/2009/07/09/09greenwire-fewer-regulations-for-bottled-water-than-tap-g-33331.html

Hans, E., & Powell, L. M. (2013, January). Consumption Patterns of Sugar-Sweetened Beverages in the United States. *Journal of the Academy of Nutrition and Dietetics, 113*(1), 43–53. doi:10.1016/j.jand.2012.09.016

High Sodium, Low Potassium Diet Linked to Increased Risk of Death: Change in Americans' Diet Necessary to Lower Risk [Press release]. (2011, July 11). Center for Disease Control and Prevention. Retrieved from http://www.cdc.gov/media/releases/2011/p0711_sodiumpotassiumdiet.html

*Importance of Water in the Diet.* (n.d.). Duke University. Retrieved from http://people.chem.duke.edu/~jds/cruise_chem/water/watdiet.html

Kline, P. (2008, May). *Question of the Month. Tap Water vs. Bottled Water: What's the Difference?* American Water Works Association. (34)5, 8-9. Retrieved from http://www.awwa.org/publications/opflow/abstract/articleid/18329.aspx

Kolata, G. (2013, May 14). No Benefits Seen in Sharp Limits on Salt in Diet. *The New York Times.* Retrieved from http://www.nytimes.com/2013/05/15/health/panel-finds-no-benefit-in-sharply-restricting-sodium.html?_r=0

Machione, V. (2013, September 18). Why Too Much Sodium Is Not As Bad As This. *Doctor's Health Press.* Retrieved from http://www.doctorshealthpress.com/food-and-nutrition-articles/why-too-much-sodium-is-not-as-bad-as-this

Malik, V. S., Schulze, M. B., & Hu, F. B. (2007, August). Intake of sugar-sweetened beverages and weight gain: a systematic review. *The American Journal of Clinical Nutrition, 84*(2), 274–288. Retrieved from http://europepmc.org/articles/PMC3210834/reload=0;jsessionid=WYsRjZV2genSm6jjC3IH.24

Mercola, J. (2013, April 4). *Why Salt Consumption Alone Will Not Increase Your Heart* Disease Risk. Mercola.com. Retrieved from www.naturalmedicine.com/news-feeds/mercola-news-feeds/why-high-salt-consumption-alone-will-not-increase-your-heart-disease-risk/

Nelson, D. E., Jarman, D. W., Rehm, J., et al. (2013, April). Alcohol-Attributable Cancer Deaths and Years of Potential Life Lost in the United States. *American Journal of Public Health, 103*(4), 641–648. doi:10.2105/AJPH.2012.301199

Osterweil, N. (n.d.). *Say it's so, Joe. The potential health benefits—and drawbacks—of coffee.* WebMD. Retrieved from http://www.webmd.com/food-recipes/features/coffee-new-health-food

Phthalate. (n.d.). Retrieved from Wikipedia: http://en.wikipedia.org/wiki/Phthalate#cite_note-CDC-4

Popkin, B. M., D'Anci, K. E., & Rosenberg, I. H. (2010, August). Water, Hydration, and Health. *Nutrition Reviews. 68*(8), 439–58. doi:10.1111/j.1753-4887.2010.00304.x

*Rethink Your Drink.* (2011, August). Center for Disease Control. Retrieved from http://www.cdc.gov/healthyweight/healthy_eating/drinks.html

Samovsky, I. (n.d.). *8 Health Benefits of Unrefined Natural Salt.* Retrieved from http://www.organicauthority.com/organic-food/organic-food-articles/himalayan-salt-an-ancient-natural-mineral-treating-todays-common-ailments.html

Silver, L., & Farley, T. (2011). Sodium and Potassium Intake: Mortality Effects and Policy Implications: Comment on "Sodium and Potassium Intake and Mortality Among US Adults." *Archives of Internal Medicine, 171*(13), 1191 doi:10.1001/archintermed.2011.271

*Sodium in Food.* (n.d.). The Food Label Movement. Retrieved from http://thefoodlabelmovement.org.2010/10/salt-part-three-changing-the-label

Sodium Intake in Populations: Assessment of Evidence [Data file]. (May 14, 2013). Institute of Medicine. *Consensus Report.* Retrieved from http://iom.edu/~/media/Files/Report%20Files/2013/Sodium-Intake-Populations/SodiumIntakeinPopulations_RB.pdf

Stolarz-Skrzypek, K., Kuznetsova, T., Thijs, L., et al. (2011). Fatal and Nonfatal

Outcomes, Incidences of Hypertension, and Blood Pressure Changes in Relation to Urinary Sodium Excretion. *Journal of the American Health Association, 302*(17), 1777–1785. doi:10.1001/jama.2011.574

Study investigates association between intake of sodium and potassium and deaths among US adults. (2011, July). *ScienceDaily*. Retrieved from http://www.sciencedaily.com/releases/2011/07/110712191650.htm

*Summary Findings of NRDC's 1999 Bottled Water Report.* (n.d.). National Resources Defense Council. Retrieved from http://www.nrdc.org/water/drinking/nbw.asp

Taylor, R., Ashton, K. E., Moxham, T., et al. (2011, August 24). Reduced dietary salt for the prevention of cardiovascular disease: a meta-analysis of randomized controlled trials (Cochrane review). *American Journal of Hypertension, 24*(8), 843–53. doi:10.1038/ajh.2011.115

Yang, Q., Lui, T., Kulina, E. V., et al. (2011). Sodium and Potassium Intake and Mortality Among US Adults: Prospective Data from the Third National Health and Nutritional Examination Survey. *Archives of Internal Medicine, 171*(13), 1183. doi:10.1001/archinternmed.2011.257

Zeiman, K. M. (n.d.). *6 Reasons to Drink Water.* WebMed. Retrieved from http://www.webmd.com/diet/features/6-reasons-to-drink-water

Zieve, D. (2012, June 23). Sodium in Diet. *MedlinePlus Medical Encyclopedia*. Retrieved from http://www.nlm.nih.gov/medlineplus/ency/article/002415.htm

# Chapter 12

Balch, P. A. (2010). *Prescriptions for Nutritional Healing* (5th ed.). New York: Avery, A Division of Penguin Group.

Beriberi. (n.d.). PubMed Health. Retrieved from http://www.ncbi.nlm.nih.gov/pubmedhealth/PMH0001379/

Beriberi. (n.d.). Retrieved from Wikipedia: http://en.wikipedia.org/wiki/Beriberi

Biotin. (n.d.). Medline Plus supplements. Retrieved from http://www.nlm.nih.gov/medlineplus/druginfo/natural/313.html

Biotin. (n.d.). Retrieved from Wikipedia: http://lb.wikipedia.org/wiki/Biotin

Calero, C., Vickers, E., Cid, G., et al. (2011, June 29). Allosteric Modulation of Retinal GABA Receptors by Ascorbic Acid. *Journal of Neuroscience, 31*(26), 9672–82. Retrieved from doi:10.1523/JNEUROSCI.5157-10.2011

*Choosing your Anti-inflammatory Supplement—What are the top picks?* (n.d.). Healthy-Diet Healthy-You. Retrieved from http://www.healthy-diet-healthy-you.com/Anti-inflammatory-Supplement.html

Chromium. (n.d.). Dietary Supplement Fact Sheet. National Institute of Health. Office of Dietary Supplements. Retrieved from http://ods.od.nih.gov/factsheets/chromium-HealthProfessional

Coenzyme Q10. (n.d.). Retrieved from Wikipedia: http://en.wikipedia.org/wiki/CoQ10

Coenzyme Q10—Topic Overview. (n.d.). Heart Failure Health Center. WebMD. Retrieved from http://www.webmd.com/heart-disease/heart-failure/tc/coenzyme-q10-topic-overview

Copper. (n.d.). Dietary Supplement Fact Sheet. National Institute of Health. Office of Dietary Supplements. Retrieved from http://ods.od.nih.gov/factsheets/copper-HealthProfessional

Copper in diet. (n.d.). *MedlinePlus Medical Encyclopedia*. Retrieved from http://www.nlm.nih.gov/medlineplus/ency/article/002419.htm

Decuypere, J. (n.d.). *Dr. Decuypere's Nutrient Charts*. Health Alternatives 2000. Retrieved from http://www.health-alternatives.com/fruit-nutrition-chart.html

Dick, J. (2013, March 5). Chlorine. Chlorine in Diet. Retrieved from https://sites.google.com/site/whatischlorine/system/app/pages/search?scope=search-site&q=Chlorine+in+Diet

Ghirlanda, G., Oradei, A., Manto, A., et al. (1993). Evidence of plasma CoQ10 lowering effect by HMG-CoA reductase inhibitors: A double-blind, placebo-controlled study. *Journal of Clinical Pharmacology, 33*(3), 226–9. doi:10.1002/j.1552-4604.1993.tb03948.x

Gordon, R. C., Rose, M. C., Skeaff, S. A., et al. (2009, November). Iodine supplementation improves cognition in mildly iodine-deficient children. *The American Journal of Clinical Nutrition, 90*(5), 1264–71. doi:10.3945/ajcn.2009.28145

Gore, J. (n.d.). *5 Signs of Vitamin Deficiencies*. Love to Know Vitamins. Retrieved from http://vitamins.lovetoknow.com/5_Signs_of_Vitamin_Deficiency

Holt, S. (2011, September 11) Vitamins and Minerals for Health Maintenance. *Holt Newsletter, 1*(11). http://www.vitacost.com/dr-holt-vitamins-and-minerals-for-health-maintenance

Hyman, M. (2012). *The Blood Sugar Solution*. New York, NY: Little Brown & Co., Hachette Book Group.

Iodine. (n.d.). Diet Supplement Fact Sheet. National Institute of Health. Office of Dietary Supplements. Retrieved from http://ods.od.nih.gov/factsheets/ Iodine-HealthProfessional

Losonczy, K. G., Harris, T. B. & Havlik, R. J. (1996). Vitamin E and vitamin C supplement use and risk of all-cause and coronary heart disease mortality in older persons: the Established Populations for Epidemiologic Studies of the Elderly. *American Journal of Clinical Nutrition, 64*(2), 190–196. Retrieved from http:// www.ncbi.nlm.nih.gov/pubmed/8694019?dopt=Abstract

Manganese. (n.d.). University of Maryland Medical Center. Retrieved from www. umm.edu/altmed/articles/manganese-000314.html

Masaki, K. H., Losonczy, K. G., Izmirlian, G., et al. (2000, March 28). Association of vitamin E and C supplement use with cognitive function and dementia in elderly men, *Neurology, 54*(6), 1265–72. Retrieved from http://www.ncbi.nlm. nih.gov/pubmed/10746596

Mercola, J. (2013, July 8). *Turmeric: The Spice That Can Potentially Help Your Health in 150 Different Ways*. Mercola.com. Retrieved from http://articles.mercola.com/ sites/articles/archive/2013/07/08/curcumin-vs-drugs-for-parkinsons.aspx

Molybdenum. (2011, April 19). American Cancer Society. Retrieved from http:// www.cancer.org/treatment/treatmentsandsideeffects/complementaryandalternat ivemedicine/herbsvitaminsandminerals/molybdenum

Murray, M. (2014, January 29). Insights Into Supplements, Nutrition and Health [Webinar]. In The Future of Nutrition Conference (January 27–31). The Institute for the Psychology of Eating.

Nourish—Micronutrients—Maintaining the Oxygen Balance in Your Brain. (n.d.). The Human Brain. The Franklin Institute. Resources for Science Learning. Retrieved from www.fi.edu/learn/brain/micro.html

Potassium. (n.d.). University of Maryland Medical Center. Retrieved from http:// www.umm.edu/altmed/articles/potassium-000320.htm

Probiotics. (n.d.). Retrieved from Wikipedia: http://en.wikipedia.org/wiki/Probiotic

Probiotics—Topic Overview. (n.d.). Digestive Disorders Health Center. WebMD. Retrieved from http://www.webmd.com/digestive-disorders/ tc/probiotics-topic-overview

Rickets. (n.d.). *A.D.A.M. Medical Encyclopedia* [Online encyclopedia]. PubMed Health. Retrieved from http://www.nebi.nlm.govpubmedhealth/PMH0001384/

Schmidt, M. A. (2007). *Brain-Building Nutrition: How Dietary Fats and Oils Affect Mental, Physical, and Emotional Intelligence*. (3rd ed.). Berkeley, CA: Frog Books Ltd.

Scurvy. (n.d.). Better Medicine from healthgrades. Retrieved from www.localhealth. com/article/scurvy

Scurvy. (n.d.). Retrieved from Wikipedia: http://en.wikipedia.org/wiki/Scurvy

Selenium. (n.d.). Diet Supplement Fact Sheet. National Institute of Health. Office of Dietary Supplements. Retrieved from http://ods.od.nih.gov/factsheets/ Selenium-HealthProfessional

Teng, W., Shan Z., Guan, H., et al. (2006, June 29). Effect of Iodine Intake on Thyroid Diseases in China. *New England Journal of Medicine, 354*(26), 2783–93. doi:10.1056/NEJMoa054022

Vitamins. (n.d.). Brianmac. Retrieved from http://www.brianmac.co.uk/vitamins.htm

Vitamins and Minerals. (n.d.). Health Check Systems. Retrieved from www. healthchecksystems.com/vitamins.html

Vitamins and Minerals: Understanding Their Role. (n.d.). Helpguide.org. Retrieved from www.helpguide.org/harvard/vitamins_and_minerals.htm

Weil, A. (n.d.). Vitamin B9 Folate. Retrieved from www.drweil.com/drw/u/ ARTO2809/vitamin-b9-folate.html

# Chapter 13

As Autumn Approaches, This Chickadee's Brain Begins To Expand; New Nerve Cells Put Fall Foraging On Fast Track. (2003, September 12). Lehigh University. *Science Daily*. Retrieved from http://www.sciencedaily.com/ releases/2003/09/030912072156.htm

Banning, D. (2013, March 13). *High but normal blood sugar levels affect brain health.* Diabetes Monitor. Retrieved from http://www.diabetesmonitor.com/education-center/high-but-normal-blood-sugar-levels-affect-brain-health.htm

Calorie Torching Workouts. (n.d.). WebMD. Fitness and Exercise. Retrieved from http://www.webmd.com/fitness-exercise/features/ high-intensity-workouts-to-burn-calories

Di Salvo, D. (2013, October 13). How Exercise Makes Your Brain Grow. *Forbes*. Retrieved from http://www.forbes.com/sites/daviddisalvo/2013/10/13/ how-exercise-makes-your-brain-grow/

Douglass, W. (2012, March 4). The silent, deadly cause of your memory problems (Hint: it's not Alzheimer's). *The Douglass Report*. Retrieved from http:// douglassreport.com/2012/03/01/cause-of-memory-problems/

Erickson K. I., Prakash, R. S., Voss, M. W., et al. (2009, October 19). Aerobic Fitness Associated With Hippocampal Volume in Elderly Humans. *Hippocampus, 19*(10), 1030–9. doi:10.1002/hipo.20547

Hellimich, N. (2013, December 13). The best preventative medicine? Exercise. *The Daily Comet.* Retrieved from http://www.dailycomet.com/article/20131230/WIRE/131239978

Hillman, C. H., Erickson, K. L., Kramer, A. F. (2008, January). Be smart, exercise your heart: exercise effects on brain and cognition. *Nature Reviews Neuroscience, 9*(1), 58–65. PMID 18094706

Ho, A. J., Raji, C. A., Beker, J. T., et al. (2011, September). The Effects of Physical Activity, Education, and Body Mass Index on the Aging Brain. Wiley Online Library. *Human Brain Mapping, 32*(9), 1371–1382. doi:10.1002/hbm.21113

Holford, P. (2007). *New Optimum Nutrition for the Mind.* United Kingdom: Piatkus Books Ltd.

Jerdziewske, M .L., Lee, V. M., & Trojanowski, J. Q. (2005, October). Lowering the risk of Alzheimer's disease: Evidence-based practices emerge from new research. *Alzheimer's Dementia Journal, 1*(2), 152–60. doi:10.1016/j.jalz.2005.09.007

Kramer, A. F., & Ericson, K. L. (2007, August). Capitalizing on cortical plasticity: Influence of physical activity on cognition and brain function. *Trends in Cognitive Sciences, 11*(8), 342–8. PBID 17629545

Lee, D. W., Smith, G. T., Tramontin, A. D., et al (2001). Hippocampal volume does not change seasonally in a non food-storing songbird. *NeuroReport, 12*(9), 1925–1928. Retrieved from http://www.ncbi.nlm.nih.gov/pmc/articles/PMC1865118/

Logan, A. C. (2007). *The Brain Diet.* Nashville, TN: Cumberland House Publishing.

Mercola, J. (2011, December 16). *80-Year Olds With 40-Year Old Muscle Mass—What's going on?* Peak Fitness. Mercola.com http://articles.mercola.com/sites/articles/newsletter-archive/2011/12.aspx

Ornstein, R., & Thompson, R. (1984) *The Amazing Brain.* Boston: Houghton Mifflin Co.

Pendick, D. (2010, Winter). Pumping neurons: exercise to maintain a healthy brain. Memory loss and the brain. In a newsletter of the memory disorders project at Rutgers University. Retrieved from http://www.memorylossonline.com/winter2010/pumping_neurons.html

Ratey, J. J. (2008). *Spark.* New York, NY: Little Brown & Co.

Renew—Exercise. (n.d.). The Human Brain. The Franklin Institute. Resources for Science Learning. Retrieved from http://learn.fi.edu/learn/brain/exercise.html

Reynolds, G. (2012). *The First 20 Minutes*. New York, NY: Hudson Press.

Servick, K. (2013, October 10). How Exercise Beefs Up The Brain. *Science Now*. Retrieved from http://news.sciencemag.org/biology/2013/10/how-exercise-beefs-brain

Shiraev, T., & Barclay, G. (2012, December). Evidence based exercise—clinical benefits of high intensity interval training. *Australian Family Physician, 41*(12), 960–2. Retrieved from http://www.ncbi.nlm.nih.gov/pubmed/23210120

Stabler, D. (2012, September 16). Move It! Living Section. *The Oregonian*, p. L1.

*The Physical Activity Guidelines for Americans.* (n.d.). 2008 Physical activity guidelines for Americans, Summary. US Department of Health and Human Services. http://health.gov/paguidelines/guidelines/summary.aspx

Vernikos, J. (2011). *Sitting Kills, Moving Heals: How Everyday Movement Will Prevent Pain, Illness, and Early Death—And Exercise Alone Won't*. Fresno, CA: Quill Driver Books, Linden Publishing, Inc.

*Walking Reduces Stroke Risk Among Women.* (2013, January 7). Medical News Today. Retrieved from www.medicalnewstoday.com/articles/254632.php

Weuve, J., Kang, J. H., Manson, J. S., et al. (2004). Physical Activity, Including Walking, and Cognitive Function in Older Women. *The Journal of the American Medical Association, 292*(12), 1454–1461. doi:10.1001/

Willey, J. Z., Moon, Y. P., Paik, M. C., et al. (2009, November 24). Physical activity and risk of ischemic stroke in the Northern Manhattan Study. *Neurology, 73*(21), 1774–1779. doi:10.1212/WNL.0b013e3181c34b58.

# Chapter 14

Alzheimer's Association. (2011). *2011 Alzheimer's Disease Facts and Figures* [Data file]. Retrieved from http://www.alz.org/downloads/facts_figures_2011.pdf

Bergland, C. (2014, February 12). Chronic Stress Can Damage Brain Structure and Connectivity. The Athlete's Way. *Psychology Today*. Retrieved from http://www.psychologytoday.com/blog/the-athletes-way/201402/chronic-stress-can-damage-brain-structure-and-connectivity

Chetty, S., Friedman, A. R., Taravosh-Lahn, K., et al. (2014, February 11). Stress and glucocorticoids promote oligodendrogenesis in the adult hippocampus [Epub ahead of print]. *Molecular Psychiatry*. doi:10.1038/mp.2013.190

Chopra, D., & Tsiaras, A. (2011, July 24). Stress and the Brain. *Huffington Post*. Retrieved from http://www.huffingtonpost.com/deepak-chopra/effect-of-stress-on-health_b_907029.html

*Chronic stress puts your health at risk*. (n.d.). Stress management. Mayo Clinic. Retrieved from http://www.mayoclinic.org/healthy-living/stress-management/in-depth/stress/art-20046037

*Coping with Stress, Injury Prevention and Control*. (2014, January). Centers for Disease Control and Prevention. Retrieved from http://www.cdc.gov/violenceprevention/pub/coping_with_stress_tips.html

DeBinder, C. (2014, April 4). Mind-Body Medicine Program Offers Meditation To Patients, Staff. *Comprint Military Publications*. Retrieved from http://www.dcmilitary.com/article/20140404/NEWS08/140409906/mind-body-medicine-program-offers-meditation-to-patients-staff

Donaldson James, S. (2013, September 12). Anxiety In Your Head Could Come From Your Gut. *ABC News, Good Morning America*. Retrieved from http://abcnews.go.com/Health/anxiety-head-gut/story?id=20229136

*Effects of Stress on the Brain*. (n.d.) DiscoveryHealth.com writers. Retrieved from http://health.howstuffworks.com/wellness/stress-management/effect-of-stress-on-the-brain.htm

Everson, S. A., Lynch, J. W., & Kaplan, G. A. (2001). Stress-Induced Blood Pressure Reactivity and Incident Stroke in Middle-Aged Men. *Stroke, 32*(6), 1263–1270. doi:10.1161/ 01.STR.32.6.1263

Geis, C. E. (2014, January). *New Stress Studies* [Data file]. Retrieved from http://www.cti-home.com/wp-content/uploads/2014/01/New-Stress-Studies.pdf

*Hans Selye's General Adaptation Syndrome*. (n.d.). Essence of Stress Relief. Retrieved from http://www.essenceofstressrelief.com/general-adaptation-syndrome.html

*How Your Brain Responds to Stress*. (n.d.). The Human Brain. The Franklin Institute. Resources for Science Learning. Retrieved from http://learn.fi.edu/learn/brain/stress.html

Klein, S. (2013, April 19). Adrenaline, Cortisol, and Norepinephrine: The Three Stress Hormones, Explained. *Huffpost Healthy Living*. Retrieved from http://www.huffingtonpost.com/2013/04/19/adrenalinee-cortisol-stress-hormones_n_3112800.html

Lupien, S. J., Schwartz, G., Ng, Y. K., et al. (2005, September). The Douglas Hospital Longitudinal Study of Normal and Pathological Aging: summary of findings. *Journal of Psychiatry & Neuroscience, 30*(5), 328–334. Retrieved from http://www.ncbi.nlm.nih.gov/pmc/articles/PMC1197277/

Parks, A. (2012, January 9). Study: Stress Shrinks the Brain and Lowers Our Ability to Cope with Adversity. *Time.* Retrieved from http://healthland.time.com/2012/01/09/study-stress-shrinks-the-brain-and-lowers-our-ability-to-cope-with-adversity/

Pickert, K. (n.d.). The Art of Being Mindful. *Time, 183*(4), 42–46.

Sanders, R. (2014, February 11). *New evidence that chronic stress predisposes brain to mental illness.* Media Relations, UC Berkeley Research. Retrieved from http://vcresearch.berkeley.edu/news/new-evidence-chronic-stress-predisposes-brain-mental-illness

Sheline, Y. I., Sanghavi, M., Mintun, M. A., & Gado, M. H. (1999, June 15). Depression Duration But Not Age Predicts Hippocampal Volume Loss in Medically Healthy Women with Recurrent Major Depression. *Journal of Neuroscience, 19*(12), 5034–5043. Retrieved from http://www.jneurosci.org/content/19/12/5034.full

Sheline, Y. I., Streeter, C. C., Jensen, J. E., Perlmutter, R. M., et al. (2007, May 28). Yoga Asana Sessions Increase Brain GABA Levels: A Pilot Study. *The Journal of Alternative and Complementary Medicine, 13*(4), 419–426. doi:10.1089/acm.2007.6338

Smith, M., Segal, R., & Segal, J. (2014, July). Stress Symptoms, Signs & Causes. Help Guide.org. Harvard Health Publications. Retrieved from http://www.helpguide.org/mental/stress_signs.htm

*Stress: Your brain and body.* (n.d.). Your amazing brain. Retrieved from http://www.youramazingbrain.org/brainchanges/stressbrain.htm

*The Effects of Stress on Memory Loss* [Blog post]. (2013, October 21). The Nerve Blog. Retrieved from http://sites.bu.edu/ombs/2013/10/21/the-effects-of-stress-on-memory-loss/

Van der Kolk, B. A., Stone, L., West, J., et al. (2013, November 14). Yoga as an Adjunctive Treatment for Posttraumatic Stress Disorder: A Randomized Controlled Trial. *Journal of Clinical Psychiatry. 75*(6). doi:10.4088/JCP.13m08561. Retrieved from http://www.traumacenter.org/products/pdf_files/Yoga_Adjunctive_Treatment_PTSD_V0001.pdf

# Chapter 15

Beta-amyloid. (n.d.). Retrieved from Wikipedia: http://en.wikipedia.org/wiki/Beta_amyloid

*Brain Basics: Understanding Sleep.* (n.d.). National Institute of Neurological Disorders and Stroke. Retrieved from http://www.ninds.nih.gov/disorders/brain_basics/understanding_sleep.htm

*Brain may flush out toxins during sleep.* (2013, October). National Institute of Health. Retrieved from http://www.nih.gov/news/health/oct2013/ninds-17.htm

Breus, M. J. (2012, August 26). Sleep Problems May Contribute to Cognitive Decline. *Huffpost Healthy Living.* Retrieved from http://www.huffingtonpost.com/dr-michael-j-breus/sleep-brain_b_1768270.html

Briggs, H. (2014, March). Lost sleep leads to loss of brain cells, study suggests. *BBC News.* Retrieved from http://www.bbc.com/news/health-26630647

Chen, A. L. (2014, April 14). More Evidence That Sleep Helps Strengthen Memory. *Huffpost Healthy Living.* Retrieved from http://www.huffingtonpost.com/2014/04/10/sleep-memory-strengthen_n_5112692.html

Devi, G. (2010, January 28). This Is Your Brain On Drugs. *HuffPost Healthy Living,* The Blog. Retrieved from http://www.huffingtonpost.com/gayatri-devi-md/this-is-your-brain-on-dru_b_439577.html

Davila, D. (2009, December). *Diet, Exercise and Sleep.* National Sleep Foundation. Retrieved from http://sleepfoundation.org/sleep-topics/diet-exercise-and-sleep/page/0%2C3/

Glymphatic system. (n.d.). Retrieved from Wikipedia: http://en.wikipedia.org/wiki/Glymphatic_system

Mann, D. (2010, January). *The Sleep-Diabetes Connection.* WebMD. Retrieved from http://www.webmd.com/sleep-disorders/excessive-sleepiness-10/diabetes-lack-of-sleep

Matthiessen, C. (2013, November 4). *Natural Sleep Aids.* WebMD. Retrieved from http://www.webmd.com/sleep-disorders/excessive-sleepiness-10/sleep-supplements-herbs

Mercola, J. (2014, April 10). *Improving Your Sleep May Be Key for Preventing and Treating Metabolic Disorders.* Retrieved from http://articles.mercola.com/sites/articles/archive/2014/04/10/sleep-deprivation-metabolic-disorders.aspx

Miller, T. (2013, June 7). Lack of sleep worsens heart disease, boosts heart attack risk by contributing to inflammation: study. *New York Daily News.* Retrieved from http://www.nydailynews.com/life-style/health/sleeping-6-hours-ups-heart-attack-risk-women-study-article-1.1366365

Prather, A., Epel, E. S., Cohen, B. E., et al. (2013, June 7). Gender differences in the prospective associations of self-reported sleep quality with biomarkers of systemic inflammation and coagulation: Findings from the Heart and Soul Study. *ResearchGate.* doi:http://dx.doi.org/10.1016/j.jpsychires.2013.05.004

Shorter Sleep Duration and Poorer Sleep Quality Linked to Alzheimer's Disease Biomarker [News release]. (2013, October 21). Johns Hopkins School of Public Health. Retrieved from http://www.jhsph.edu/news/news-releases/2013/spira-sleep-alzheimer.html

Sleeping Pills: What You Need to Know. (2006). WebMD. Retrieved from http://www.webmd.com/sleep-disorders/features/sleeping-pills-what-need-know

Spira, A. P., Gamaldo, A. A., An, Y., et al. (2013, December). Self-Reported Sleep and β-Amyloid Deposition in Community-Dwelling Older Adults. *The Journal of the American Medical Association Neurology, 70*(12), 1537–43. doi:10.1001/jamaneurol.2013.4258

What is Sleep? (n.d.). American Sleep Association. Retrieved from http://www.sleepassociation.org/index.php?p=whatissleep

Whiteman, H. (2013, October). *Lack of sleep may increase Alzheimer's risk.* Medical News Today. Retrieved from http://www.medicalnewstoday.com/articles/267710.php

Xie, L., Kany, H., Xu, Q., et al. (2013, October). Sleep Drives Metabolite Clearance from the Adult Brain. *Science, 342*(6156), 373–377. doi:10.1126/science.1241224

# Chapter 16

Cohen, S., Alper, C. M., Doyle, W. J., et al. (2006). Positive Emotional Style Predicts Resistance to Illness After Experimental Exposure to Rhinovirus or Influenza A Virus. *Psychosomatic Medicine, 68*, 809–815. Retrieved from http://repository.cmu.edu/cgi/viewcontent.cgi?article=1272&context

Cole, S. W. (2009, June). Social Regulation of Human Gene Expression. *Current Directions in Psychological Science, 18*(3), 132–137. doi:10.1111/j.1467-8721.2009.01623.x

Cole, S. W. (2012). The Science of Compassion: Origin, Measures and Interventions. In Conference Presentation: Telluride, CO, July 19–22. Published on August 27, 2012, by CCare at Stanford University. Retrieved from http://www.youtube.com/watch?v=ZCqYMdYa5DY

Dixon, A. (2011, September 6). *Kindness Makes You Happy—And Happiness Makes You Kind*. Greater Good: The Science of a Meaningful Life. Retrieved from http://greatergood.berkeley.edu/article/item/kindness_makes_you_happy_and_happiness_makes_you_kind

Fratiglioni, L. (2004, June). An active and socially integrated lifestyle later in life might protect against dementia. *The Lancet Neurology, 3*(6), 343-353. doi:10.1016/51474-4422(04)00767-7

Fredrickson, B. (2013). *Love 2.0: How Our Supreme Emotion Affects Everything We Feel, Think, Do, and Become*. London, England: Penguin Book Ltd.

Gregoire, C. (2013, August 23). The 75-Year Study That Found The Secrets To A Fulfilling Life. *HuffPost The Third Metric*. Retrieved from http://www.huffingtonpost.com/2013/08/11/how-this-harvard-psycholo_n_3727229.html

Healthy You. (2013, December–2014, January). *AARP The Magazine*, p. 16.

Kiecolt-Glaser, J., McGuire, L., Robles, T. F., & Glaser R. (2002). Emotions, morbidity, and mortality: New perspectives from psychoneuroimmunology. *Annual Review of Psychology, 53*, 83–107. Retrieved from http://www.ncbi.nlm.nih.gov/pubmed/11752480

Li, S., Jin, M., Zhang, D., et al. (2013, March 16). Environmental Novelty Activates β2-Adrenergic Signaling to Prevent the Impairment of Hippocampal LTP by Aβ Oligomers. *Neuron, 77*(5), 929–941. Retrieved from http://dx.doi.org/10.1016/j.neuron.2012.12.040

Mahoney, S. (2012, December). How Love Keeps You Healthy. *Prevention*. Retrieved from http://www.prevention.com/sex/sex-relationships/how-love-keeps-you-healthy

Marchione, M. (2013, July 6). Study: Retiring later lowers dementia risk. *The Oregonian*, p. A1 & A4.

Moskowitz, J., Epel, E., & Acree, M. (2009). Positive affect uniquely predicts lower risk of mortality in people with diabetes. *Health Psychology, 27*(1), S73–S82. Retrieved from http://psycnet.apa.org/journals/hea/27/1S/S73/

Ornstein, R., & Sobel, R. (1987). *The Healing Brain*. New York, NY: Simon & Schuster.

Rowe, J. W., & Kahn, R. L. (1998). *Successful Aging*. New York, NY: Random House.

Steptoe, A., & Wardle, J. (2005). Positive affect and biological function in everyday life. *Neurobiology of Aging, 26*(1), 108–12. Retrieved from http://www.ncbi.nlm.nih.gov/pubmed/16213629

Vaillant, G. (2008). *Spiritual Evolution*. New York, NY: Broadway Books, Random House, Inc.

Wilson, R. S., Krueger, K. R., Arnold, S. E., et al. (2007). Loneliness and Risk of Alzheimer Disease. *Archives of General Psychiatry, 64*(2), 234–40. Retrieved from http://www.ncbi.nlm.nih.gov/pubmed/17283291

# Index

283

# About the Author

KAREN V. UNGER, M.S.W., ED.D., IS AN EDUCATOR AND AUTHOR with a lifelong interest in health. She has a background in psychology, social work, and education, and has worked for three decades in the fields of mental health and education. Initially motivated by a report about the poor health of people within the Oregon Mental Health System, Dr. Unger began a four year project to understand why so many of us have become unhealthy and what we could do about it.

Using her extensive experience in research and education, she has brought together the latest information on the underlying causes of our current state of health and on how we can prevent disease and vastly improve not only our general health but our brain health as well. *Brain Health for Life* is the result of that project.

She has written a previous book, book chapters, peer-reviewed articles, federal policy papers, and an *Evidence-Based Practice Kit for Supported Education*. While at Boston University, she was a senior staff person at the Center for Psychiatric Rehabilitation and an adjunct professor at Sargent College of Allied Health Professions. She has also been a research associate professor at the Community Rehabilitation Division, Arizona State University in Tucson and is currently a research associate professor at the Graduate School of Education at Portland State University. Dr. Unger is president of Rehabilitation Through Education and lives in Portland, Oregon.

For more information visit brainhealthforlife.net or brain-healthforlife.net/blog.

CPSIA information can be obtained
at www.ICGtesting.com
Printed in the USA
FSOW01n2222091214
3723FS